Title: Enjoy The Journey

Author: Rodney Washburn

ISBN: 9798584476618

Version 1.3 – December 2020

Published by Rodney Washburn at KDP

Discover other works by Rodney Washburn at www.rodneywashburn.com

This short book is a work of non-fiction. The names, characters and incidents are all real.

This book is dedicated to my mother.

TABLE OF CONTENTS

INTRODUCTION

I want to sincerely thank you for purchasing this short book, <u>Enjoy the Journey</u>! I have thoroughly enjoyed my journey, and I want you to have a similar experience and success. I am a big believer in data driven processes and I think I have clearly laid out one here for you. I am confident that if you follow the process as designed, you will see positive results. This is a logical process that works, and as other diet fads come and go, I am sure it will stand the test of time. I am also looking forward to receiving feedback from the reviews of this publication to improve future versions. So please, whether you love it or hate it, take a few minutes to leave me your comments. Also, the Excel spreadsheet I developed to go along with this short book is included with this purchase and can be found at: https://rodneywashburn.com/the-books/.

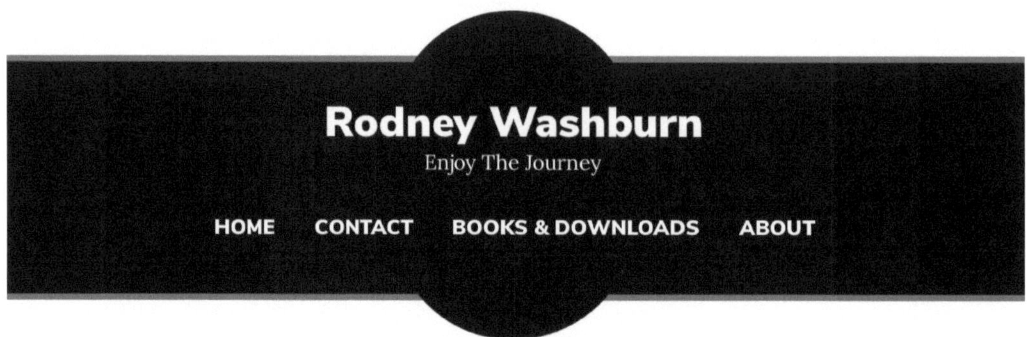

Hello world! Thank you for visiting! I am using this site to provide links to all my published works and downloadable supplements.

RODNEY'S FACEBOOK PAGE

Framing the Problem

My target audience is anyone seeking to lose weight that has yet to find the right process that works for them. Being overweight makes people suffer from low self-esteem and feelings of inadequacy. If you are reading this, it is most likely because your weight is affecting you negatively, curtailing your enjoyment of life, and potentially damaging your health. Millions of people worldwide wake up every day and walk around with a nagging feeling about their weight. They are insecure about it and frequently wear certain outfits to cover it up. They lack the confidence to wear a bathing suit at the beach or wear clothes highlighting their body's physical features. This was how I was living, and it was a miserable feeling. I wasn't unhappy, but it was something that bothered me immensely.

I grew up living an active lifestyle as a teenager and then joined the Marines after high school. Being physically fit was easy in those days. Working out was enjoyable and I could keep my weight down while eating whatever I wanted. After the Marines, I began a career in law enforcement. I was still single and volunteered for active assignments like the bike patrol to stay fit. Having no family responsibilities, I would spend hours in the gym several times a week lifting weights before or after my shifts. I was so active that I would literally eat fast food twice a day and maintain low body fat percentages.

Then I got married and became a father in my early thirties, so my priorities shifted. The new responsibilities cut into my exercise regimen. I also moved up into the management ranks at work, which took me off the bike patrol. My family became the central focus in my life, and exercise became something I would only do sporadically when I had time. The problem with all this was that I maintained my high-calorie diet, and over the years, I began adding on weight.

The weight gain was a gradual process that transformed my body over about ten years. During that time, I would go through dieting and exercise periods, but any progress I made was only for a few months. My experiences were a pattern of temporarily losing weight, then gaining it back, and usually with a few additional pounds. After an extended series of this "yo-yo" dieting, I felt that sustainable weight loss was not achievable. Soon I began telling myself that it was just part of the aging process and that I should accept my body as it was and be happy. I did this for years, yet I could never shake the feelings of failure or unhappiness I felt from the constant reminder of this defeat, and it left me feeling inadequate. I would see other men and women my age that were in great shape. They worked out, wore form-fitting clothes, or would take pictures on a beach in a bathing suit. They were everywhere on social media, and it made me feel envious. I said I didn't want to be them, but I found myself avoiding taking pictures because I hated what I saw. I have an entire decade of my life with my kids while growing up where I rarely had pictures made because it hurt too much to see what I had become.

Things began coming to a head for me at the end of 2019. I had just turned 48, and at 5'9", I weighed well over 200 pounds. I was the clinical definition of obese, and it was a miserable feeling. I hated the way I looked and I wanted a change, but I was afraid I would fail again. I bought some weights and started working out, but my joints hurt. I was falling apart. I couldn't run anymore because my knees ached. I tried dieting here and there, but nothing seemed to work. I had no willpower. I started carrying a journal around with me and logging what I ate in a food diary, and it seemed like it was helping, but nothing dramatic or worth mentioning. Then in March 2020, I went to the doctor for a sinus infection. When I arrived, the nurse asked me to take off my shoes and stand on the scale. I assumed the reading would be somewhere around 212, because, in my mind, that is what I thought I weighted. That was what I saw when I looked in the mirror at home. Then I stood on the scale. I was floored when the reading came out at 230 pounds. I was completely and utterly devastated. I don't remember anything else from that day, just the feeling of being a failure again.

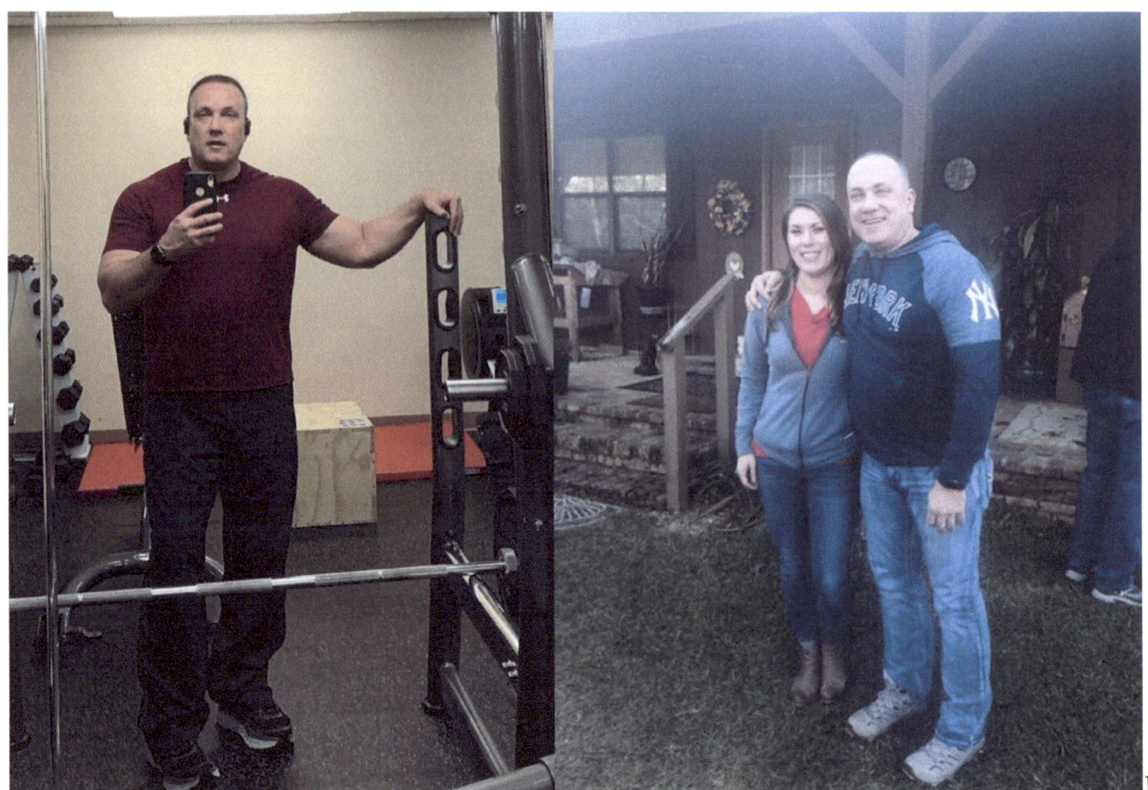

Pictures of me from July 2019, and then again in November 2019 at 230 pounds

I went back home that day and just sat and thought about this issue for a bit. Then I took off my shirt and looked at myself in the mirror. Then I took a few pictures of myself from several different angles, and it was shocking what I saw. The reality of how bad things were truly hit home, and it was not a good feeling. But then something happened.......I got mad.

I have always been successful in life at whatever I set my mind to accomplishing. I felt like I could do anything I set out to do, except this. This is the one area of my life where I felt like a failure, and it was creating doubt in my abilities in other areas of my life. I realized right then and there that if I didn't beat and overcome this, I would always feel like a failure. I also realized that if I could overcome this problem, it would set me on fire to accomplish challenging goals in other areas of my life. This was the fight of my life. If I beat this, I could do anything. But how?

According to the World Health Organization, 14 percent of the world's population is overweight, and in the United States, that figure is a staggering 40 percent. A quick search on Google revealed that there are thousands of diet plans, schemes, books, and products. The diet industry is a multi-billion dollar industry supported by millions of people seeking solutions to their weight gain. This research made one thing clear: Losing weight is tough. It is very tough. Obesity is one of the biggest problems plaguing a large portion of the population. It's so severe that many people have given up and just accepted that they cannot change their body composition and strive to be happy as they are. But at the same time, I knew this wasn't the way it had to be. There were clear signs of others making it, and living happy, fulfilled lives in a healthy, strong body. They live active lifestyles, look great in their clothes, exude confidence, and appeared to be very happy. That was where I wanted to be.

My first step of this journey began with framing the problem: Accurately identifying the relevant variables to maximize weight gain or loss. As I mentioned earlier in the book, I started a law enforcement career after leaving the military. I am now in my 25th year of that career. I have had a very successful career and have held a wide variety of command and leadership positions at all organization echelons. My current assignment is serving as the Chief of the Data Science Division. I was tasked with standing up a data science capability and then overseeing all data science operations. I also have vast experience in intelligence operations, requirements development, acquisitions, and asset allocation procedures. I say all of this only to highlight that over the years, I have gained a great understanding of planning, gap analysis, requirements development, systems engineering, resource deployment, advanced analytics, and the scientific method. It was through this lens of experience that I approached this problem. In other words, I decided to make this a research project that would entail properly framing the problem, and then developing an in-depth analytical approach to understanding the problem, capturing what is known, and then developing a hypothesis to test and record what works and what doesn't.

Once I decided to approach it in this way, it was just a matter of following the process, conducting the analysis, recording the results, and then making further adjustments until I achieved the desired results. This process is the significant achievement of this study.

The Process

In addition to the experience above, I also have a passion for college football. I am a fanatic! I love it! And having grown up in Alabama, I am a diehard Auburn fan. If you are familiar with this region of the country, you know that football is akin to a religion in the state. It is not uncommon to hear about houses being divided over the rivalry between the Alabama Crimson Tide and Auburn Tigers. No matter who you are in the state, you must pick a side. However, I have not lived in the state for over three decades, so I can look at things more objectively. My career has led to a love of processes, so when Nick Saban became the Alabama football team's head coach, I perked up. I am still a diehard Auburn fan, but I am also a student of Nick Saban's "The Process."

In discussing the process, Nick Saban commonly refers to not focusing on the long-term goal that is months away, or even the short-term goal of what you want to achieve this week, but rather an intense focus on the current task at hand. The process entails developing a long-term strategic desired end state, and then intermediate goals and objectives. But success comes from the minute to minute battle within yourself. Your process has to detail what you must do every minute of the day to be a success. You then follow the process from minute to minute, and if properly designed, it will lead you to your short-term and long-term goals.

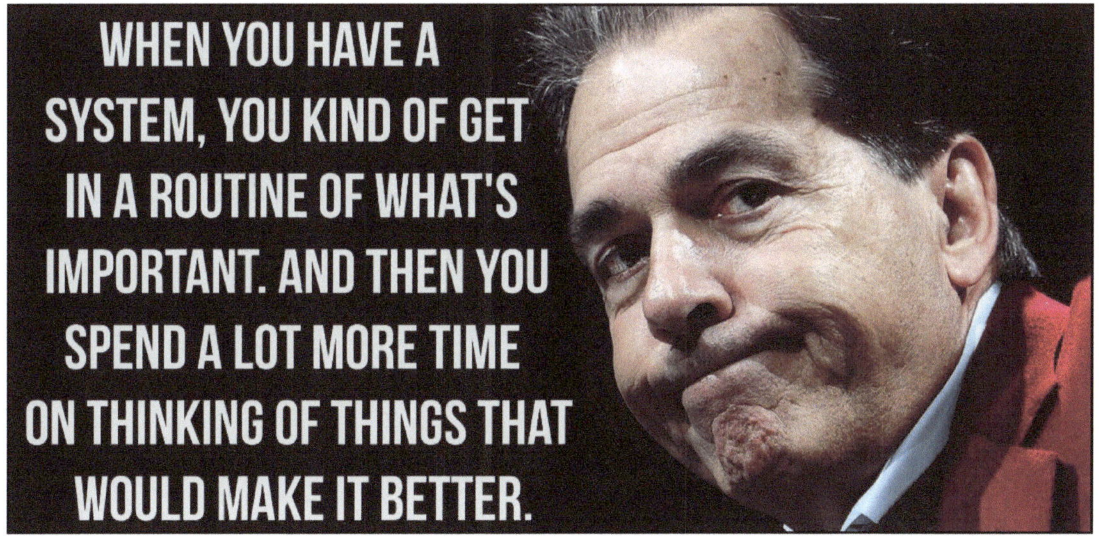

For football players at Alabama, each player has a structured process that they follow each day. Throughout the day, they only focus on what they are currently working on and being the best they can be at the moment. In the games, the players do not focus on the scoreboard, but instead being the best they can be for the play happening right now. If they can achieve success on each play, more often than not, the score will take care of itself. By focusing on this process, Nick Saban has built a powerhouse program that is a routine contender for the national title each year and has made him arguably one of the greatest coaches in college football history.

Through my study of this "The Process," I came to understand several principles that remain near and dear to me. Everything in life is a process, but most are not clearly defined or coherent, so the fruits of the process vary. However, the successful ones are clearly defined, easy to follow, but difficult to adhere to. In other words, the path is clear, but success entails raising your standards and getting outside of your comfort zone. Sound processes demand you maintain a focus on results to achieve your goals and objectives. So my research would focus on what works and then incorporate that into a clearly defined process that I could follow each day, leading me to achieving my desired results over time.

My Results

What you are reading now is the process I developed over my weight loss journey. The journey was hard, and there were many times I felt incredibly frustrated. But once I found what works through trial and error, I was able to layer these components into an overall process that made weight loss a fascinating journey.

I also need to say that I am not a certified personal trainer or fitness guru. I do data science. I used this knowledge to conduct my experiment on myself, and these are the findings.

Here are some of the achievements I am most proud of:

- A loss of 40 pounds of fat while maintaining my muscle mass (from 230 to 190)
- A reduction in body fat from 35% to 15%
- My waist, as measured to the largest circumference of my gut, was reduced from 45 inches to 35 inches (in jeans went from a size 36 to a size 32 in the waist)
- My shirt size went from an extra-large to a medium
- I can run again! Daily! And for long distances! Up to 7 or 8 miles.
- I have clarity and understanding of how my metabolism works, and I know without any doubt how to dial my diet in to maintain a desired weight
- I feel happy, confident, and in complete control of this aspect of my life

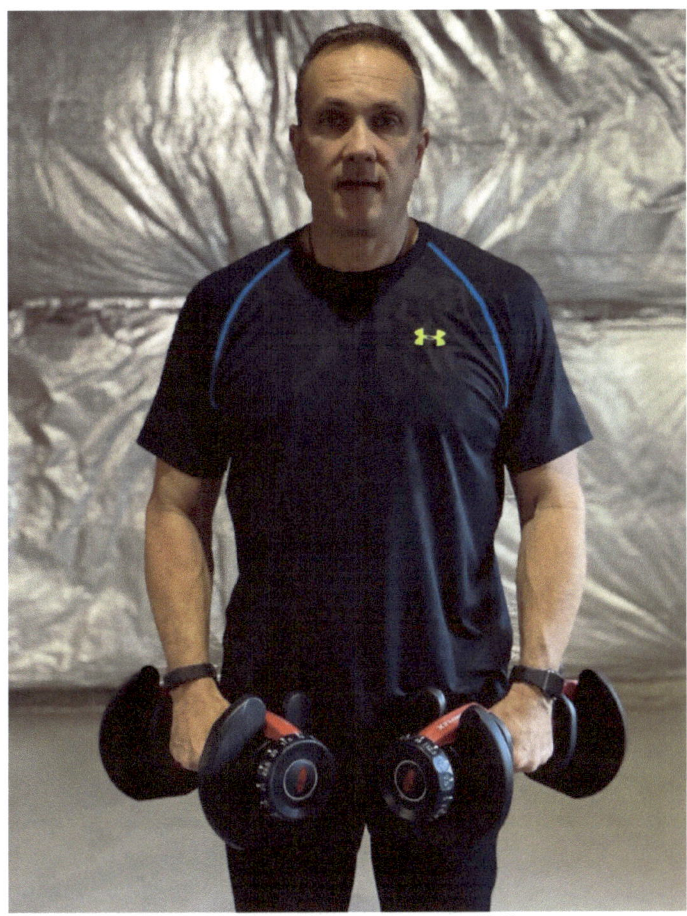

Feeling much better now at 190!

Most of all, I now feel unstoppable, like there isn't anything I can't do. I am confident that if applied with discipline and perseverance, it will work for you as well! Over the next few chapters, I will layout the key concepts that I discovered that really worked. I will show you how to set up your own step-by-step process to guide you through each day that only requires focusing on the immediate time frame. This focus will help you accomplish your goals. I will also explain what data you need to track and consistently document. This data is the feedback loop that will tell you if what you are doing is working or not. Capturing the right information is imperative to the process because it will tell you almost immediately if what you are doing is working or not.

Action Leads to Motivation

I cannot adequately convey how completing this journey will change every aspect of your life. Doing so will open your eyes to seeing what is truly possible once you set your mind to something. There is great reward in developing a plan of attack and sticking to it until you achieve your goals. It is truly one of the most rewarding things you will ever do and the fruits of your labor will be present each day when you get dressed and look in the mirror. You will love seeing you again! So without further ado, let's begin.

CHAPTER ONE: NEURO-LINGUISTIC PROGRAMMING

The Strongest People are not those who show strength in front of us, but those who win battles we know nothing about. – Jonathan Harnisch, "The Brutal Truth"

My journey began on December 31, 2019. That is the day I hit rock bottom. New Year's Eve and I was depressed. I was fat and disgusted with my inability to lose weight. I had dieted most of the previous year but to no avail. I was fatter than ever. I had tried low carb, no-carb, Paleo, Keto, you name it, but I was a complete and utter failure. What frustrated me most was that weight loss is framed as a simple math equation and willpower, right? Burn more calories than you consume, and you will lose weight. I knew this to be accurate, yet I failed, and I couldn't understand why. So that night I resolved again, to lose weight.

I started researching weight loss programs on the Internet, but not in the traditional sense. I had already lost faith in the fad diets. See, I understood how the math works in regards to weight loss. What I did not understand was why I couldn't maintain the negative calorie balance that led to weight loss. I always started the day with good intentions, but once the day wore on and hunger set in, I would inevitably fail. I wanted to understand why, and I knew the problem was in my head. My failure was more than a lack of will power, so I dug in.

- <u>Frame the Problem</u>: Inability to maintain a disciplined diet.
- <u>Symptoms</u>: I would start each day out with a diet plan and good intentions. I could make it through most of the day, but then I could barely maintain my meal plan for diner when I got home at night. I would come off the rails! I would experience uncontrollable urges. I knew it was wrong, but my willpower would collapse, and I would eat large quantities of prohibited foods. I would then feel a sense of tremendous guilt for having failed again.
- <u>Question</u>: Why do some people fail where others succeed? Is it merely willpower, or is there something more sinister at work here? It felt like my brain was overwhelming my ability to maintain control and was betraying my desire to eat a healthy diet.
- <u>My Research</u>: Could Neuro-Linguistic Programming, also commonly referred to as NLP, teach me to more effective communications with my brain?

What is NLP?

NLP was developed in the 1970s by Richard Bandler and John Grinder. They started down this path by asking why some people achieve results where others do not. I was asking myself the same thing! Why do some people go on a diet and have tremendous success at losing weight, and then others go on the same diet and lose none, or worse, gain weight? While the question may seem simplistic on the surface, it is incredibly profound and thought-provoking. They found that two people could have the same education and training, yet success was determined by how successful they were at communicating, either with others or themselves. Bandler and Grinder found that successful people do things in quite the opposite manner than those who are unsuccessful, and thus was born the concept of NLP.

In more simplistic terms, NLP is how to program your mind to work for you and not against you. The brain seeks short-term pleasure, even at the risk of suffering from longer-term damage. Sure we know that a cigarette may kill us, but in your twenties, the risk of dying in your fifties from lung cancer seems a long time away, so you smoke for the short-term pleasure and discard the risk of longer-term pain. You know you need to quit, but the short-term pleasure you derive from smoking outweighs the longer-term desire to stop. That is because the benefit felt from smoking is felt immediately, whereas quitting would be painful. From a logical standpoint, you will feel much better overall from not smoking, but the pain you feel while trying to break your addiction is overriding your will to resist the need for that short-term pleasure. This is why quitting is so hard, and yet, some people do stop. Is it more manageable for some to resist the temptation to smoke than others?

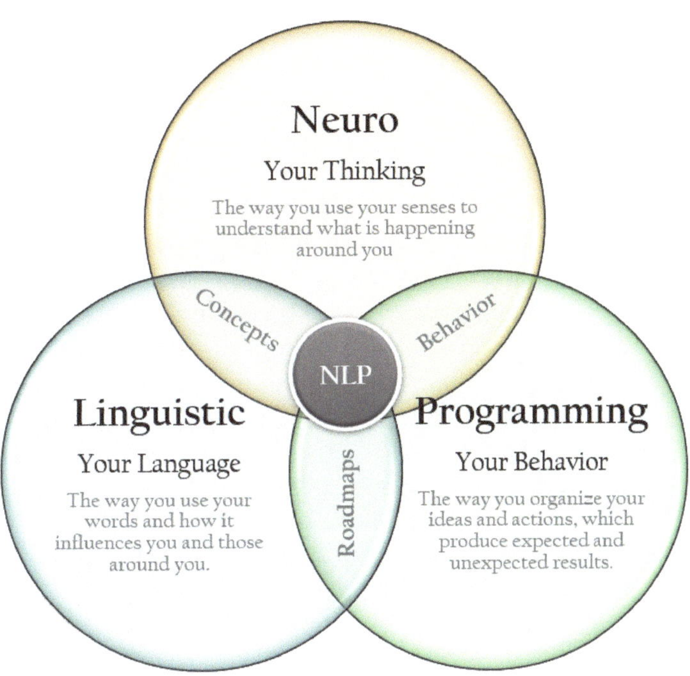

This same concept can be applied to anyone who procrastinates from doing anything that would be better for them in the long-term. Avoiding doing whatever you need to do – clean the house, mow the yard, etcetera – is less painful than actually doing it. Then we feel the pain of regret, guilt, and a sense of being a failure. This is a mighty force in our minds, and the people that achieve success have a better mastery over it than those that don't. This is why you start the day out with great intentions to eat healthy foods, like a low-calorie dressing on your salad, and end up with a double cheese burger. You get hungry and your mind wants you to feel pleasure, so it generates the cravings for the tasty food that is the worst possible choice you could make, yet the urge is so powerful that it overwhelms you to give in. Before you know it, you have swallowed the burger and feel a sense of guilt for failing. Many people feel the guilt but haven't analyzed why they failed. They shrug it off, and if they feel defeated, they may stop the diet they just started because it is simply too difficult. Others try to get back on the wagon the next day only to fail again by noon. Meanwhile, they have that co-worker that comes in looking great, and at lunchtime, whips out that salad with grilled chicken and a low-calorie dressing and enjoys it like it is the best thing they have ever eaten. It makes you sick, envious, and even resentful.

After researching NLP, I knew this was an area I needed to explore. I went straight to the best: Tony Robbins. Tony Robbins started teaching NLP techniques in the 1980s and quickly became recognized as one of the best at teaching people how to reprogram their minds. On his site, Tony Robbins advertises at 10-day weight loss program that focuses on sustainable weight loss strategies to transform your health. As I reviewed the literature, I felt like Tony was talking to me when he said, "Willpower by itself is not enough; if we want to achieve lasting change, we must have an effective strategy." I purchased it immediately and started the 10-day course on New Year's Day.

One of the main concepts of NLP is that people who are more successful than others, when everything else is equal, comes down to how they communicate with their brains. Once we have ingrained a habit into our programming, overwriting that programming can be incredibly challenging to do, but it is not impossible. Everyone can do it, no matter the habit or addiction, it just takes understanding and effort. You must come into this with a positive mindset. Even if you have failed repeatedly, you must come into this with certainty that you are starting on the path to success.

Through my self-reflection, I realized that I had failed so much at dieting that I had reached a place called "learned helplessness," and nothing I tried would work. Learned helplessness is a condition in which a person suffers from a sense of powerlessness from a traumatic event or persistent failure. It is also thought to be one of the underlying causes of depression, which makes logical sense. It occurs when an individual continuously faces a negative, uncontrollable situation and stops trying to change their circumstance, even when they can do so. We see this with people that try to quit drinking, smoking, and dieting. I have come to believe that the fat was permanent and that all I could do was accept it. Once you buy into this belief, you are done!

To break the chains of this illogical belief required some intense soul searching and focus on what I wanted to achieve. Whether it's consciously or subconsciously, whatever we focus on is what we will get. So I started an intense focus on what I wanted to achieve. Here is the goal I set for myself:

> **Goal:** Lose half a pound of fat per week until I reduced my body weight from 230 pounds down to 190. From there, I would reassess my goals and objectives to see if I wanted to go to 175 pounds. At 190 pounds, the mirror, or more specifically, my abs, would be my guide that determines if I needed to lose more. I wanted to see clearly defined abs within twelve months.

SMART Goals

Just a brief mention of SMART Goals. Goals give us a sense of direction, motivation, a clear focus, and clarify importance. Your goals are the target you are aiming for; however, most people do not set realistic goals, or they are ambiguous. For this reason I highly recommend ensuring you use SMART Goals: Specific, Measurable, Achievable, Realistic, and Time Bound.

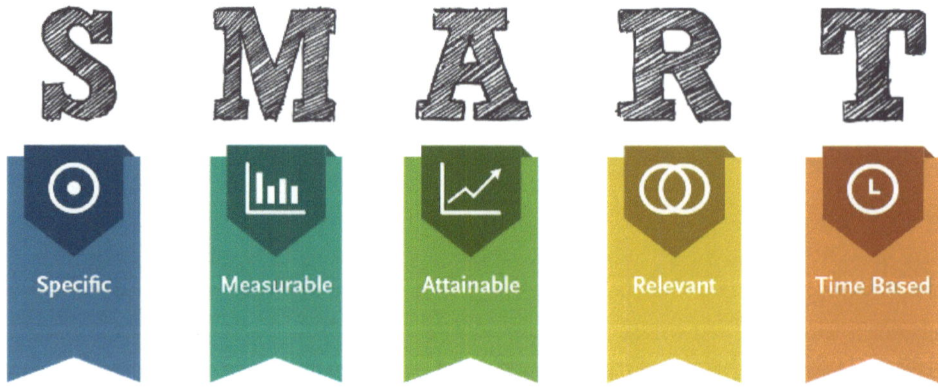

- <u>Specific</u>: What is it exactly that you want to do? For me it was lose 40 pounds of fat while maintaining muscle mass.
- <u>Measurable</u>: How will you measure success? I wanted to lose the 40 pounds of fat, reduce the circumference of my gut by 10 inches, and run again.
- <u>Achievable</u>: Do you have the resources and capabilities to achieve these specific and measurable goals? For me it was do or die. If I did not achieve it I was going to be a miserable human being forever, and that was not acceptable.
- <u>Realistic</u>: Are your goals realistic? We are only human, so we need to be realistic in what we want to achieve. I knew I could lose weight, but making my hair grow back was off the table.
- <u>Time Bound</u>: Your goals need to be time based. My goal was to lose half a pound of fat per week, so with a goal of 40 pounds, I knew it was going to take 90 weeks to get there by losing half a pound a week.

Based on my estimations it seemed like a long time, but then I realized it was a lot of weight to lose, and I surely didn't get this fat overnight, so I shouldn't expect it to be gone overnight. I liked the plan because half a pound of fat a week seemed reasonable, and I felt confident I could handle it. I committed to staying focused and accepted that there would be setbacks. When setbacks and trying times occurred, I made a serious commitment to staying the course. I also committed to having open conversations with myself at night around dinner time when I was the most vulnerable to cravings. When the desires came, I would talk to myself about how I felt and why I was feeling this way.

Overall the results were mixed. Sometimes I failed and gave in, but over time I became more successful at walking away. One trick I learned was that a short brisk walk around the block would often kill my cravings. This started interrupting the programming my mind had written, and I began to win the battle of will over my cravings. I knew I wanted to enjoy myself and the body that God gave me. I wanted to look physically attractive and live with a sense of vitality. To date, that desire to change had been met with pain and failure, but no more. I was on the path of developing a strategy that revolved around a process that would keep me focused and committed to losing the weight.

Furthermore, I accepted that I had to take responsibility for losing the weight and that I alone would have to do all of the work required. This created new empowering patterns that I then focused on programming into my brain as a permanent part of my life. Lastly, I committed to enjoying the journey. I believed that if I could make some initial progress, it would motivate me to progress further. Success would beget success. Here are some bullets outlining where I maintained a focus for NLP efforts:

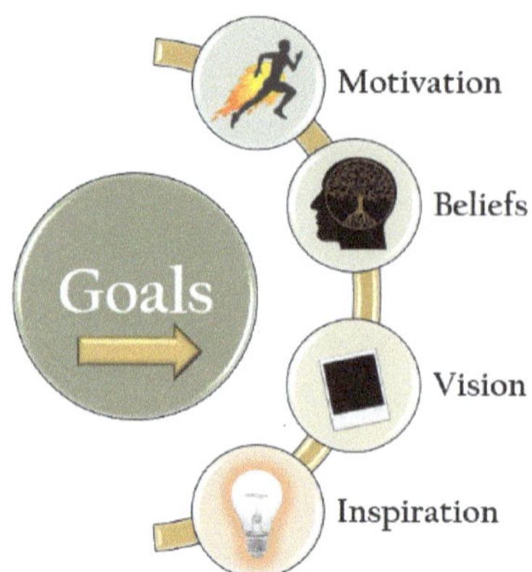

- <u>Get in the Right Frame of Mind:</u> Make change a must. Find leverage and motivation to make it happen. Mixed emotions were holding me back. I was unhappy, yet I was not making the sacrifices required to make the changes I desired. My survival instincts programmed to avoid pain told me to lower my standards and accept how I was, but I refused to believe the problem was permanent.
- <u>Challenge Limiting Beliefs</u>: I began actively identifying the limiting beliefs holding me back and challenging them. I determined that I had suffered long enough and that it was time to make a real change.
- <u>Develop a Vision:</u> I identified my end state in terms of how much I wanted to weigh, and a visual of what I wanted to see in my abdominals.
  - <u>Changed My Wardrobe</u>: I would not allow myself to buy any more new clothes for my current weight. Extra-large shirts were tossed out, and I only kept large shirts in my closet. If I wanted a new shirt, I had to buy in size medium and let it sit until I could fit into it. I also kept these new shirts I wanted to wear in view for motivational purposes and would try them on from time to time to see how I was progressing.
  - <u>A Picture Is Telling</u>: I kept a picture of what 40 pounds of fat looked like on my phone and posted one in my office so I could see it frequently. I also took pictures of myself without a shirt from the front and side. I would pull these pictures out when I was having discussions with myself over cravings at night. Many times it was the deciding factor that helped me win the battle over the cravings.
- <u>Find Inspiration:</u> I identified things in my life that would remind me why this was so important to me. This included missing out on the joys of life and being a good role model for my kids.
  - <u>Missing Out</u>: I made a list of all the areas of life I was missing out on because I was disgusted with myself. This included: not going out with friends, not going to the lake or beach, and not wearing stylish clothes. Overall it was having a severe impact on my self-esteem.
  - <u>Set the Example</u>: I decided I wanted to be an example for my kids to follow. Several times over the last few years, I wondered if my weight embarrassed my kids. They never said so, but I am sure at some level they were because I was. How were my low standards regarding my weight impacting them?

Although this strategy worked for me, the results were limited. I realized that this would just be one of the tools in my toolbox required to lose the weight. But the experience was invaluable in understanding the power of the mind and learning how I could communicate with myself to win the battles over it to achieve the results I desired. NLP is effective as a part of a comprehensive process, but not as a standalone method.

Is NLP Right For You?

I touched on NLP here only to introduce it as a concept that I focused on to change my bad snacking habits. It worked for me, but it is not a silver bullet. If I had to quantify it, for me, it was good for about five pounds initially. NLP is best taught by people with in-depth study in the subject matter and there are many options out there. I recommend Tony Robbins only because I like him and his approach has worked for me. I am not an NLP expert, so I do not want to make it look that way. But I do believe our minds work against us in ways we do not always fully understand. Abraham Maslow famously stated, "What is necessary to change a person is to change his awareness of himself." That is what NLP did for me, and I think if you approach it with an open mind, you will gain a greater understanding of many of your negative behaviors in life.

Key Takeaways

I started this chapter out with a quote by Jonathan Harnisch describing the challenges of overcoming the subconscious mind. If you are like me, when I started down this path, you are probably feeling like a failure and couldn't understand why. This chapter is just one small piece of the puzzle, but hopefully, you have gained some awareness as to "why" you fail, which makes you feel this way. The problem is not a lack of self-discipline, but rather a need to reprogram the communications between what you desire and how you behave. NLP is a real thing, and today there are many different options for consumers to choose from. You will need to do some legwork to identify what behaviors and triggers you need to change, but NLP offers a real path forward towards doing so. I am partial to Tony Robbins because of the clear and concise manner his courses are laid out, but you can go with whoever works best for you.

Develop an end-state vision and set realistic goals. I put my goal at half a pound a week because I felt it was reasonably achievable. I also gave myself a reasonable time frame to get there. Two years may seem like a long time, but I was determined to make a life change, and so I was ok with making slow progress so long as it was positive progress. Lastly, don't let failure get you down. You can lose the battle but still win the war. Get back after it when you experience a setback. Make setbacks motivating forces. Do not let them turn the tide of the war. Decide what is important to you by finding reminders that will inspire you to keep going. Find ways of staying focused on your daily process.

This simple awareness of how I was communicating and interacting with my brain was tremendous progress for other areas of my life as well! I realized that many triggers were signaling me to act counter to my desires and self-interest. I already knew that willpower was not enough, but understanding how I had hardwired my brain into taking specific actions and then practicing reprogramming it was invaluable, showing me the realm of what is possible. I hope you understand that your mind is like a software program for a computer, and it is written to force you to take specific actions. You are not failing so much as you are merely doing what your brain has been programmed to do. This is why you fail at your short-term attempts to diet. Weight loss through sheer willpower will come back with a vengeance. Sheer willpower causes mental exhaustion, so even if you achieve your goals, you will wake up a few months later and find the fat has returned. Reprogramming is vital to long-term success.

When cravings come on strong, you must remember that the brain's primary goal is to duplicate the experience of pleasure and avoid the experience of pain in the immediate time frame without any consideration for the future. This is why procrastination is so prevalent in our society. The longer you avoid the near-term discomfort for a longer-term pleasure, you keep re-enforcing the program, making it even more potent. This reprogramming will not be easy. The brain will resist, so you have to focus on these limiting patterns and continuously override them until you succeed. Remember, unhealthy foods generally taste great, and therefore give you a sense of pleasure. The pain of gaining weight is perceived as distant, so the brain does not feel a sense of pain from the thought. You must also remain alert for triggers that create a desire to eat. A sense of scarcity causes urges that lead to binges. There seems to be some addictive property to simple carbohydrates, like potato chips and cookies that draw you in when you go a stretch without food. You may not always win, but becoming aware of them is the start of understanding that will lead to change. Your mind is always seeking pleasure and inviting you to eat. This is the biggest obstacle you will need to overcome, and success will require planning and preparedness. Remember, this is a war, so if you lose one battle, regroup and keep fighting. Don't give up! Reassess why you failed, and take actions to improve.

You are what you eat! So in the next section, we will start discussing diet. I will cover what I found in my research and what worked for me. After that, we can discuss my research on fitness and exercise, and I will cover what worked for me. After that, I will get more specific about diet and macros, and then I will cover how my process unfolded. The last section will walk you through setting up your plan.

Chapter Two: Actions And Support Tools

There are two pains in life. The pain of discipline and the pain of disappointment. If you can handle the pain of discipline then you'll never have to deal with the pain of disappointment. – Nick Saban

There is no one right way to lose weight. It is a process, and that process has to be supported by specific steps and many of these steps require support tools. The mathematics is to burn more calories than you consume, but there are many ways to approach how you can do that. My process lasted months, and over that time, I experimented with many different concepts and techniques to find what worked for me. The diet and weight loss industry is so large that it can be difficult to parse through all the crap products to find what is real and what isn't. I tried many different tools and concepts out, discarded most, and then fine-tuned the ones that worked to suit my temperament, lifestyle, and focus. In other words, I know what I can and cannot do, so I had to ensure my approach was practical. What follows are some of the things that worked for me.

Food Diary

On January 1, 2020, I began keeping a food diary of everything I put into my mouth. Initially I purchased a nice leather-bound journal for logging everything. I thought I had a good idea of how much I was consuming, but the results were shocking. It was immediately apparent that I was eating mindlessly without any awareness of the types and amounts I was shoving down my gullet. I committed to logging everything and quickly became annoyed with catching myself grabbing a handful of nuts or a piece of candy off someone's desk, and then having to pull out my log and write it down. There was also a strong temptation to mentally write off that piece of candy and justify it as "only ten calories," but I was committed. What saved me was the sense of disgust I felt with myself, so not logging it would only make me feel worse. Pulling out the log and writing it down only to have people ask me what I was doing was a little embarrassing, so my commitment to doing so gave me the strength to start passing on some of these snacks. After logging my meals for a few days, I reviewed it and was shocked at how much I was consuming, especially my coffee consumption. I was downing five or six cups a day. Add in the creamer (35 calories per tablespoon) and it was a lot of extra calories.

This approach was enlightening, but to be honest, I did not lose a lot of weight. I did gain a disturbing awareness, but this alone did not move the needle much, so I had to go back and reassess my efforts. I cut down to three cups of coffee per day, and I limited snacking, but since the fat was not falling off, I decided to reassess and fine-tune my process. Looking over my logbook, I decided to get more precise with my portions sizes, caloric consumption, and measuring serving sizes. An accurate depiction of what I was consuming was the order of the day.

Fitness Apps

My first step was the MyFitnessPal app by Under Armor. I had it for a long time, but never really used it. MyFitnessPal is one of the most popular web-based exercise and fitness social media applications available. You can use it to track your daily food and beverage intake, calculating all your nutrients, calories, and vitamins. The free app is sufficient for what you need, but I upgraded to the premium version to perform better analysis. The app is excellent for many reasons, but my favorite feature is the bar code scanner that provides a breakdown of your macros per serving from packaged foods in seconds. This is great because it makes the data capturing and input easy to do, which gives you a greater chance of success. After all, your tracking is only as good as the data you provide for the analysis. The adage in data analysis regarding information is "garbage in, garbage out." The developers of this app put a lot of emphasis on convenience during development.

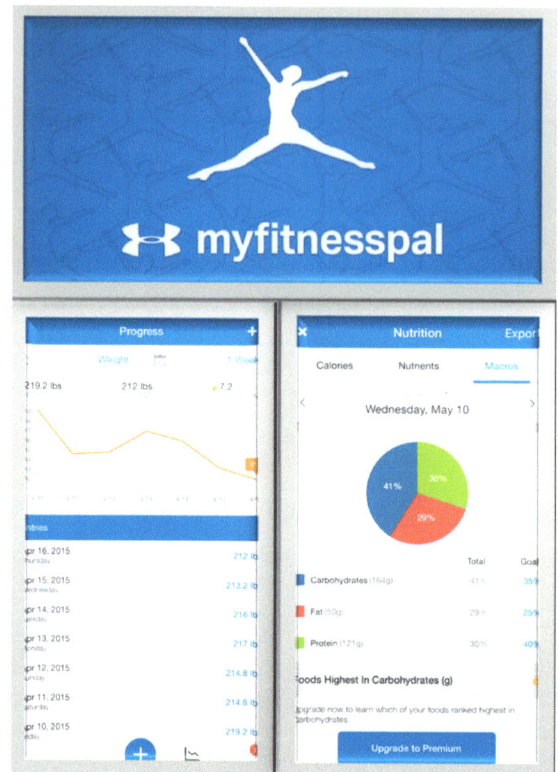

One quick note on using fitness apps to track calories. Most apps will baseline your calories burned per day based on the data you provide regarding your age, height, weight, and activity levels. This is what it says you burn on a regular day, not counting your workouts. You will need to baseline this by consuming the recommended number of calories and seeing if your weight goes up or down. If you are tracking it accurately and it stays the same, then you are dialed in. If you start gaining weight, then you will need to reduce the number of recommended calories. We will get more into that in chapter 4, but the point is this: the app makes a recommendation, but you will need to dial it in based on what the data is telling you.

Also, many of these apps will default to add in the calories burned while working out to the total calories you have available to eat. So if you usually eat 1800 calories per day and burn an additional 300 calories while working out, it will add these calories to your 1800, giving you 2100 calories to consume. While this may make dieting more comfortable, it may also make you fatter. Turn this default off. If your target calories are 1800, stick with 1800. Don't compensate by adding them to the total or not while you are in fat loss mode. Once you reach your target weight goal, you may want to experiment with it, but track it closely and turn it off again if it leads to unwanted weight gain.

Food Scale & Measuring Cups

A mechanism for accurate tracking is essential, but just as vital to your efforts are accurate weights and measurements of food consumption. Before I purchased a scale and some measuring cups, I thought I was eating correct portions sizes. Boy, was I wrong! I was serving myself way too much! My estimations of a fist-size serving, or what was a teaspoon of spread, were way off. The result was I was eating about 400-500 calories per day more than I thought I was. This was skewing the data and ruining my analysis – garbage in, garbage out.

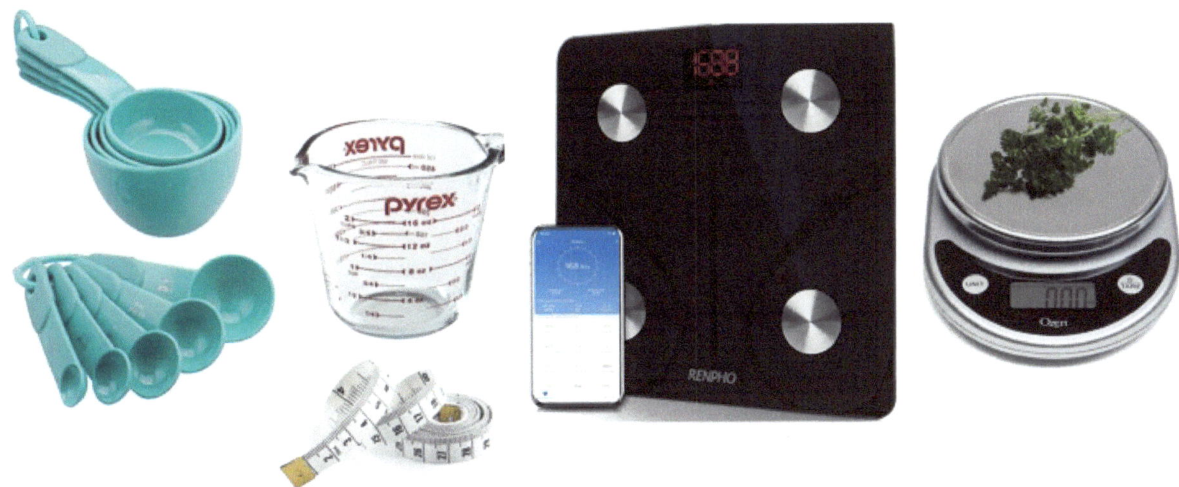

My experience is common, which is why you need to invest in the right tools. Research studies confirm that most people underestimate their portion sizes, especially for high-calorie foods such as nuts, butter, spreads, sauces, and salad dressings and toppings. I also found that when I was hungry, I would routinely miscalculate portion sizes to a greater degree. Seeing the disparity in my assumptions about serving sizes made this a significant advancement in my process. It is probably one of the critical factors that have contributed the most to my success because of the accuracy it provides your diet.

I purchased various sizes of measuring cups for my kitchen to measure anything whenever I needed to have confidence that I had the measurement right. I also bought a small digital food scale for about $22. It has been tremendous and has given me confidence when measuring my food servings to feel confident in the data. It also keeps me from consuming more calories than intended. Once you start using measurement instruments, you will quickly see how using the eyeball method can easily go over your assumption by 100 calories or more. It also takes the subjectivity out of the size of fruits and vegetables.

The measuring cups will assist you in accurately capturing things like a cup of strawberries or vegetables. You cannot underestimate the impact this type of tracking will have on your overall results. Losing fat comes down to a caloric deficit, and that requires precision if you want to drop about 200 calories a day from your diet. I have also found that it has taught me what a portion is for all sorts of food I commonly eat, so when I go out to a restaurant or something, I can make an educated guess on portion sizes. When I was having trouble losing fat, I started measuring everything, and it worked! I even started calculating how much coffee creamer to use, my butter when cooking, and especially my salad dressings. And even though I am much better at eyeballing the amounts, I still use my measuring cups and scales religiously. I also started using smaller plates for the psychological aspects of having a large amount of food on my plate.

The last piece of this process was cutting boards and knives. I was eating more fresh vegetables, so I made sure I had four or five cutting boards and small knives at the ready to slice and dice my veggies as needed.

Tape Measure and Weight Scale

I purchased a scale for capturing my weight that tracks things like BMI, muscle mass, and body fat percentage. Now I am aware these scales are not precise, but the data outputs are consistent, so I found them useful for gauging progress. As a part of my process, I initially started weighing myself upon waking every Saturday morning, but later on, I added a weigh-in day on Tuesday. Twice a week worked well for me because I am aware our weight fluctuates day-to-day, so instead of becoming routine, I made it a twice a week check-up. I would weigh myself on Saturday, and by Tuesday, if I were not making progress, I would reassess my efforts and see where I needed to tighten things up.

The tape measure was only used to measure the circumference of my stomach. My gut was what annoyed me about being chubby. I hated the way I looked, especially how it protruded from my shirt, even when covered. At the start of my weight loss journey, the largest part of my gut measured 45 inches around. Today, as I write this with a 35 measurement in the same place, the amount of fat loss is mind-boggling.

Key Takeaways

I want to reiterate what I said at the beginning of this chapter; losing weight is a process. Your process will involve using tools in a toolbox to aid your weight loss efforts, and when and how they are applied is what makes up your process flow…or routine. I will set you out on the process I followed, but since there is no one right way to lose weight, you will tweak it towards what works best for you. However, your tweaks must be supported by data, which will be derived on Saturdays and Tuesdays when you check your weight and take your measurements.

One of the best tools in your toolboxes is a food diary because of the awareness it provides. You will have the most interaction with your food diary because you will be utilizing it every time you eat, so it is a core part of the process. I prefer MyFitnessPal because I am familiar with it, so it's merely a personal preference. There are other options, so shop around and find one you like and will use. Handwritten journals are ok, but the functionality of app-based trackers is hard to beat, especially when you can use the barcode to scan in serving size and immediately track your macros (more on macros in chapter 4).

A food scale and measuring cups are vital to your success! Do not discount the impact these tools will have on your results. They are very affordable and you will save money in the long run because they will ensure you are eating the proper serving sizes. We will baseline the number of calories you require daily to maintain your current weight and then we will scale your caloric intake back by 200-300 calories per day. This will keep you from feeling like you are starving. It is incredibly easy to overestimate serving sizes and portions and one daily mishap could hamper progress.

Lastly, you will need a tape measure and a weight scale. You will use the tape measure to take quick measurements of your problem areas twice a week. I was only tracking my gut's circumference because that was the part of my body that disgusted me the most. You may want to measure your upper arms, neck, hips, thighs, or whatever bothers you. I do not recommend measuring everything. You could, but you want the process to be quick and efficient. After you take your measurements, you will get on your scale and capture your weight. I bought an excellent scale and downloaded an app that goes with it. It captures my body weight, body fat percentage, muscle mass, and BMI.

In the next chapter, I will discuss my exercise regimen. Like everything else involved with weight loss, there is no one size fits all. I will share my experiences and what worked for me, and then you can tailor your plan and then track the data to see what works for you. The following chapters will get more specific about diet and macros and then I will cover how my process unfolded. The last section will walk you through setting up your plan.

CHAPTER THREE: EXERCISE

What you get by achieving your goals is not as important as what you become by achieving your goals. – Henry David Thoreau

As I began this journey, I had some anxiety about exercise. I was always physically active when I was younger, but I found that my joints hurt more and more when I would go out and move as I aged. This was especially true for my knees and shoulders. In my mind, I told myself this was part of the normal aging process, but it was still nagging at me inside. My joints would ache with any form of physical exercise and I found myself saying that I just could not run anymore because my knees hurt. Mentally I chalked it up to my age, but then I would see someone much older than me running and it didn't make sense. I started doing some research, and there was one nagging question I did not have an answer for: Could my knees hurt when I run because I am too heavy? Had I gotten so fat that it hurt my joints to carry my weight around? I was 48 at the time and I would see marathon runners in their 60s. It just didn't make any sense. So I made this one of my research questions:

Do my joints hurt no matter what, or would the pain ease over time and weight loss?

I wanted to approach this problem and find a solution that would not cause me so much discomfort that I dreaded my workouts. I wanted to enjoy pain free exercise again. With this in mind, I set out to design a walking routine that would gradually ease into a running routine. I also began lifting weights again.

Weights

Working out with weights was something I enjoyed since I was a teenager. I always appreciated how it made me feel and how it could quickly transform your body. Lifting has always been a personal challenge for me. Early on, I adopted the habit of logging each workout by sets, reps, and how I felt. I note when I feel like I could do more weight by jotting down a recommended attempt weight for my next lift. My past experience gave me a pretty good idea of how to get back into the weight room. I started out focusing on just a few sets of moderate-to-heavy weight of 5-to-7 reps for 3-to-5 sets. I used my log to maintain an ever-increasing intensity with either more weight or additional reps. If this is not a habit for you, I highly recommend you adopt it. Otherwise, you could spend months in the gym and become discouraged with a perceived lack of progress that could easily be avoided.

My basic weight lifting routine only takes about 20-30 minutes to complete and leaves me feeling pumped and satisfied. I only dread getting started, but once I warm up, I feel great. I had not lifted weights for some time, so I felt some incredible joint pain when I first started back. At first, I chalked it up to old age but enjoyed the feeling in my muscles when I was done, so I kept at it. The pain was terrible and would sometimes wake me up at night. Over time I found that extra warm-up sets and stretching exercises before lifting heavy did help a lot. I also used heat-inducing creams on my shoulders to get the blood flowing, which also helped reduce the pain. It was incredibly discouraging at first, but over about seven months the pain went away. Now I warm-up and lift with hardly any pain at all. So what I thought was old age setting it was just cobwebs from lack of use. Once my tendons and ligaments strengthened, the pain went away. So don't be discouraged if you feel pain. Warm-up thoroughly and keep at it. It does get better!

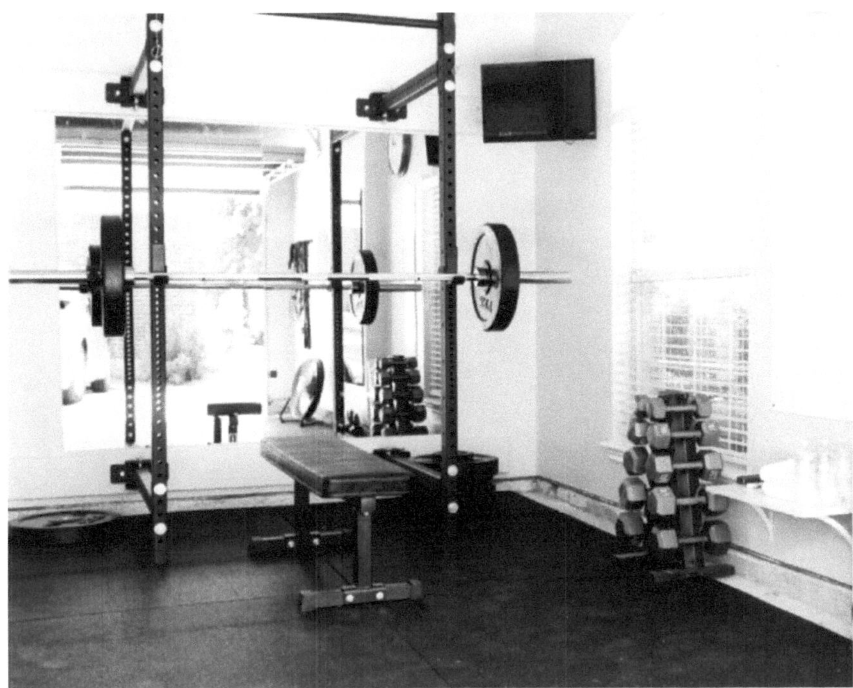

Here is an example of my weightlifting routine for chest and triceps.

Flat bench barbell press:

- Warm-up set: Lift the 45-pound bar for two sets of 10 repetitions
- Lift 135 pounds for two sets of 10 repetition
- Lift 185 pounds for 1 set of 4 repetitions
- Lift 235 pounds for three sets of 5-7 repetitions

I maintain intensity against my muscles either through an increase in repetitions on a set or an increase in weight. I do this by taking a weight, say, 100 pounds, and doing my three sets. If I achieve seven repetitions on all three sets, I will increase the weight by five or ten pounds and drop my repetitions down to four or five, and over the next few weeks, work my way back up to seven. Once I reach seven on all three sets, I start all over again. I do variations of this for all of my weight workouts, and keep all of them about this short. For back and biceps, as another example, I do pull-ups with weights with the same concept, and then do shoulder shrugs, and then bicep curls. For legs, I mainly focus on the leg press. Squats still hurt my knees quite a bit, and with age now, my hips feel like they wants to pop out, so I find workarounds. I say all of this to mean: find what works for you, a workout you enjoy, and be happy and stick to it.

Walking

My initial cardio regiment revolved around walking. My knees hurt too much to run, and while I suspected the pain was from being so heavy, I wasn't sure. So I decided to begin with a focus on walking. I wanted to be somewhat ambitious, so I set a daily goal of 15,000 steps per day. To get after this, I scheduled a walk in the morning and a walk in the evening. These two walks, coupled with whatever walking I did during the day, usually hit the mark. My first walk of the day was always two miles. My second would be as far as it took me to reach my 15,000 daily step goal. I also added in tricks to get more steps, like parking in a parking lot 1-mile from the office or parking on the far side of the parking lot when I went to the store. Little tricks like these, or taking the stairs instead of the elevator, really do add up. I frequently did short walks around the neighborhood that do not require much strength or stamina. I also found short walks would kill any cravings that popped up for sweets throughout the day. If you get an urge, go for a walk, and it may eliminate it.

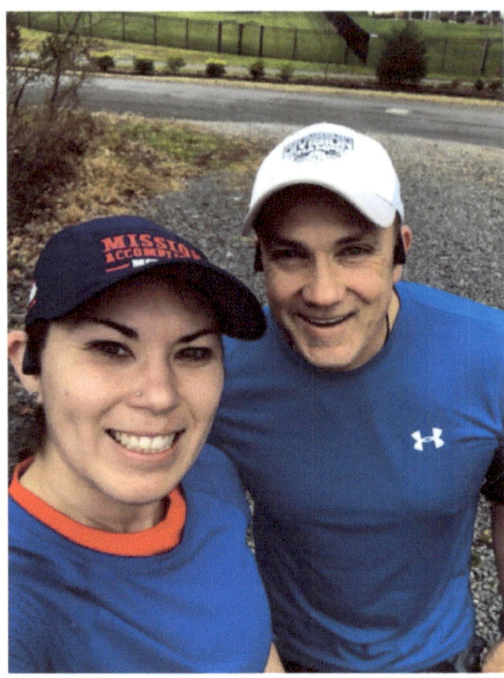
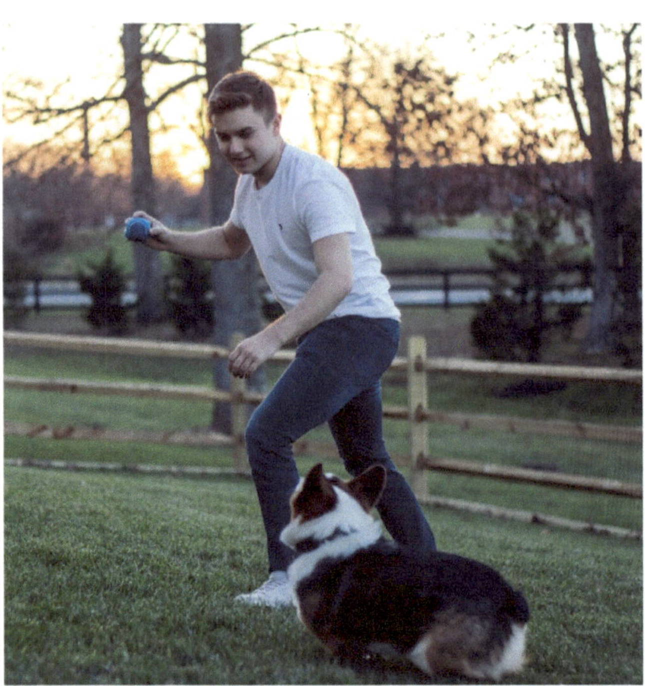

Fitness can be a family event

A funny thing happened when I started this regiment: the dog got healthier too! I would always take the dog on these walks, and boy, did he love it! In the evenings, my kids would join in, and we would have some lovely family discussions while strolling around the neighborhood. It was great! Walking is a great low impact way to kick off your foray back into fitness. Now that I have achieved my desired weight, I modified my daily goals to burn 1,000 move calories per day. I track this on my Apple watch, but I am sure Fitbit and other popular fitness trackers have similar features.

Running

My venture back into running was not smooth, but it wasn't as bad as I thought it would be. After walking for a few months, I was ready to attempt running, albeit with some anxiety over the coming knee pain. My first stop on this journey was the local running shoe store. I wanted to make sure I consulted with some knowledgeable and experienced runners and got a high-quality shoe. I went with the Hokas and have never looked back!

While I was at the running shoe store, I told the manager that I had not run in over a decade with any consistency and was concerned about knee pain. He recommended an app called "Couch to 5k" on the Apple app store. It is made by Zen Labs and is focused on beginning runners. I downloaded the app and gave it a try, but admittedly abandoned it after two weeks. The app had me progressing along, but I wanted to take things a little slower, so I used the same concept, but my

own design. I made me a playlist on my smartphone of about fifty songs I wanted to run too.
Additional information on this approach can be found by studying the "Galloway Method[1]" of run-walk intervals to build your base.

In the first few weeks, I would run one song and walk one. I would do this for two miles.
After two weeks, I started running two songs and walking one, again doing this for two miles. I
would change my route up daily, and the variance in the length of the songs changed the intensity
from day-to-day. For example, on one day the two songs may only total six minutes, and the next
time I would run, it could take eight minutes. It all depended on which songs were selected, which I
had set to random. After another two weeks, I ran three songs and walked one and eventually
worked my way up to four songs. At four songs I dropped the program and just continued running
for various distances that ranged from two to five miles, depending on how I felt that day. I would
have knee pain the following day after a long or intense run, but nothing like I thought I would
have.

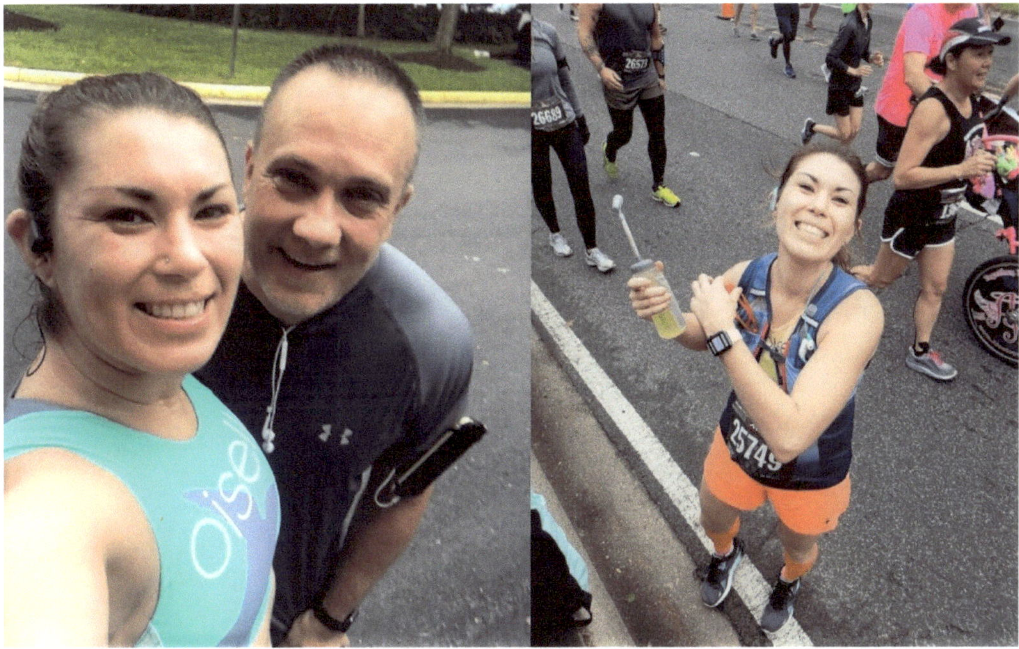

Running with my partner in crime August 2020 – Ashley is an avid runner, which helps me a lot!
(Left: Running in the neighborhood, Right: Ashley running the Marine Corps Marathon)

Being able to run again was a game changer! I love the feeling of smoothly moving along the
path and feeling my breath. The intensity is based strictly on how I feel. I am more focused on
having fun than competing, and nothing feels better than completing a run. I am grateful for this
experience and glad that I took the time and effort to get back into running because it does lift my
mood. When I was younger, I was always focused on time and distance when running, but now I
love the feel of being out there and doing it. It is incredible, and if you think you cannot get back
out there, I urge you to think again. I thought my running days were over, but now I believe they
are just beginning. I plan to run into my senior years and I will love every mile of it.

---

[1] *The Galloway Run-Walk Method", Jeff Galloway*

Key Takeaways

Transitioning from a sedentary lifestyle to an active one can induce anxiety, especially if you are overweight. It is easy to chalk it up to aging and accept a lower standard, but that nagging feeling of how it makes you feel will not go away, which is why you are here. When I began my journey, I was concerned about joint pain hindering my ability to exercise, but it got more comfortable and more enjoyable over time. There will be a period at the beginning where your joints will be sore, but as your ligaments and tendons strengthen, the pain should subside. Some of the remedies that worked for me were thoroughly warming up and applying a cream like Icy Hot to areas like my knees and shoulders.

Your workouts should be focused on increasing your strength, muscle mass, and improving the cardiovascular system. For me, this was a basic weightlifting program and running. For you, it may be something else that you enjoy. But whatever you choose, do it with sufficient intensity to do the job. Walking is a great way to exercise on your rest days because it is so low impact that it doesn't hurt your body. It will energize you and make you feel more alert. I initially set my step goal at 15,000 steps, but now that I run almost daily, I focus on obtaining 1,000 move calories daily. When you start running, find a running program that works for you, but more than anything, make it enjoyable. This will ensure you look forward to and will continue to exercise. If you find yourself dreading your workout, scale back on the intensity (And don't skimp on the running shoes!).

In the next chapter, I will cover diet, macros, and intermediate fasting. Then I will cover how my process unfolded. The last section will walk you through setting up your plan.

CHAPTER FOUR: DIET

Success will continue only as long as the commitment to the process of being successful remains in place. – Nick Saban

When it comes to losing weight, it doesn't matter if you go low carb, no-carb, high carb, or something else, but rather that you burn more calories than you consume. It is that simple. However, if you want to maintain your muscle mass while reducing body fat, the quantity and quality of the calories consumed are critical. This does not mean you have to starve though, because quality foods can be made to taste great!

When I started this journey, I set a goal of losing a pound of fat per week. My rationale was that this should be achievable and sustainable. There are 3,500 calories in a pound of fat, so mathematically, this means I would have to figure out how many calories I burned per day, on average, and then reduce it by 500 calories (3,500 divided by seven days in the week). This was more than I anticipated, so I also considered losing only half a pound a week, which would reduce my caloric intake by 250 calories per day. In the end, I went with 250, but the point is you can do it either way. However, if you go with 250 calories, you need to make sure you accurately calculate the number of calories you are consuming. With that decided, I set out to operationalizing this into my daily process.

Baselining Your Total Daily Energy Expenditure (TDEE)

Now I know I said that a loss of one pound of fat per week mathematically requires a reduction of 3,500 calories, but it is more complicated than this. Losing weight is hard to do, and that is why so many of us feel dejected. The reality is that this process will impact each of us differently and with a variety of outcomes. Overall, this process can be tracked, monitored, and adjusted to dial your weight into where you want it to be. I recommend focusing your diet on whole natural foods and eating more healthy meats like chicken and fish. If there are foods in your house that will hurt your diet, throw them out now. If it is there, and it tempts you, you will eat it when you get hungry.

Once you decide how much fat you want to lose per week, you have to baseline your total daily energy expenditure. What is this? Your total daily energy expenditure, commonly referred to as TDEE for short, is the total number of calories your body burns daily. To burn fat, you must eat fewer calories than your TDEE. Doing so will force your body to use fat for fuel. There are dozens of free TDEE calculators on the Internet, or you can create your own in a spreadsheet (e.g. Microsoft Excel). This is only a starting point because if you are consistent in tracking your caloric intake, then the data will speak for itself rather quickly, allowing you to dial-up or down as needed.

Your Base Metabolic Rate (BMR), or your metabolism, is the number of calories required to keep your body functioning at rest. The formula uses the variables of height, weight, age, and gender to calculate your BMR. This is more accurate than calculating calorie needs based on body weight alone. Note: BMR is similar to the Resting Metabolic Rate (RMR), and the two are sometimes used interchangeably.

These are foundational calculations for you because, from them, you will start monitoring how many calories a day you need to maintain or lose weight.

Harris-Benedict BMR Equation

The Harris-Benedict Equation formula uses your BMR and then applies an activity factor to determine your total daily energy expenditure (calories). This equation will be very accurate in all but the very muscular and the very fat.

Here is the formula:

Women	BMR = 655 + (4.35 x weight in pounds) + (4.7 x height in inches) - (4.7 x age in years)
Men	BMR = 66 + (6.23 x weight in pounds) + (12.7 x height in inches) - (6.8 x age in years)

Your Total Daily Caloric Needs (Total Daily Energy Expenditure - TDEE)

Once you have your BMR, you will then determine your total daily caloric needs by multiplying your BMR by the appropriate activity factor based on your lifestyle:

Sedentary (little or no exercise)	Calorie Calculation = BMR x 1.2
Lightly active (light exercise/sports 1-3 days/week)	Calorie Calculation = BMR x 1.375
Moderately active (moderate exercise/sports 3-5 days/week)	Calorie Calculation = BMR x 1.55
Very active (hard exercise/sports 6-7 days a week)	Calorie Calculation = BMR x 1.725
Extra active (very active and physical job)	Calorie Calculation = BMR x 1.9

So if you are currently sedentary, multiply your BMR by 1.2. For example, if your BMR were 1,800 calories per day, your total daily caloric needs would be 1,800 X 1.2 = 2160 calories per day. This is the total number of calories you need to maintain your current weight. This should be a relatively accurate measurement of your TDEE.

This is a starting point for determining your daily caloric needs. There is also the Kate McArdle equation, but it really isn't necessary because you will know how many calories your body needs to maintain its current weight once you start tracking the data.

Your Daily Caloric Needs for Fat Loss

Once you know the number of calories needed to maintain your weight, you can easily calculate the number of calories you need to eat to gain or lose weight. You can shave off as few as 250 calories per day, or be more ambitious and go for 500. Both will work so long as you are accurately capturing your caloric consumption. If it isn't working, then the problem will most likely be either:

- You need to reduce your caloric intake further, or
- You need to improve your tracking of the data, which means you are not correctly weighing and measuring your food portions

In the beginning, it is imperative that you accurately measure your portions, weigh your food, and log your meals. Plan your meals so that your daily caloric intake does not exceed your goal, determined by how much fat you want to lose per week. If you are failing to stay within the confines of your goals, then the problem is either:

- You are being too ambitious and need to dial back the caloric reduction to lose less fat per week, or
- You need to focus on you NLP to understand better why you are not true to yourself

I recommend starting with NLP first. Your mind is not on your side here.

Once you have accurately tracked the data for a few weeks, you will see if the calculation maintains your current weight, causing you to gain weight or lose weight. You can even see how much. If you gain a pound of fat, and you know that you are accurately capturing your caloric intake, then you would do this:

- A pound of fat is 3,500 calories
- That equates to 500 calories per day
- You must cut 500 calories from your calculated TDEE to accurately depict your total daily caloric needs to maintain weight
- Try it for a week, see what happens, and reassess

This is the starting point. By accurately tracking everything you eat, you will develop a level of self-awareness that you previously never had. If you record the data in a spreadsheet, or some other way, like an app, you will know in a matter of weeks how many calories you are consuming, and the impact that is having on your weight. If your weight increases and you can see the fat coming on, you are consuming more calories than burning. If your weight is dropping, then you are burning more than you are consuming. My point to all this is to say that you will soon learn what your TDEE truly is by tracking the data.

Setting Your Macros

Up to this point, we have focused on caloric intake. Incorporating macros goes one step further by tracking the ratio of macronutrients you consume in terms of grams of proteins, carbs, and fats. This is where we dial in the quality of the food you consume. When I started tracking my macros, I set the goal of maintaining my muscle mass while I lost the fat. Why? Simply because I didn't want to be one of those who looks sickly and thin because they dieted all their muscles away. I wanted to maintain my muscle mass so that I would look fit, strong, and healthy. To do so, I started calculating my macros by focusing on protein intake.

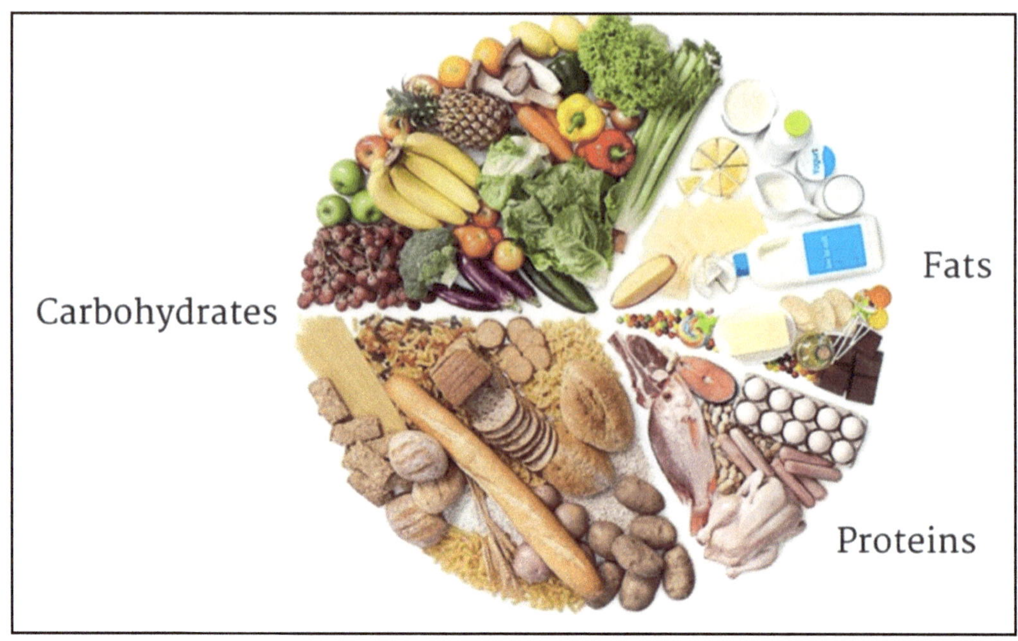

Protein

Muscles need protein to grow. I wanted to ensure that I was getting sufficient protein in my diet that my body would have ample muscle growth from my workouts while allowing it to burn body fat. I am not a doctor, but to me, this just seemed logical, so I tried it. I estimated that I would need 1 gram of protein per pound of bodyweight daily. At the time, my TDEE was around 2,300 calories, and fat loss was accelerating between 1,800-1,900 calories. So I used 1,850 as my daily caloric baseline.

- Example body weight = 200 pounds
- TDEE = 2,300
- BMR = 1,850

So to determine the grams of protein I needed daily I used the following equation:

- 200 pounds x 1 gram of protein = 200 grams of protein per day
- Each gram of protein contains four calories
- 200 grams of protein x 4 calories = 800 calories
- Breakdown:
    - 800 of my daily 1,850 calories must come from protein
    - That leaves 1,050 for fat and carbohydrates

Fat

In researching the proper percentage of calories that should come from fat, there was no concise answer, but most of the sources I read recommended 20-25 percent of your daily calories coming from fat. There was no clear answer why, so I decided to go with 25 percent. I went with 25 percent simply because each gram of fat has nine calories, so it would be challenging to eat healthy fats with my meals while keeping it at 20 percent of my calories. There is no science behind my determination, just my own logic.

I determined the grams of fat I needed daily by using the following equation:

- Fat = 25 percent of daily caloric intake
- Daily caloric intake equals 1850 (my BMR)
- 25 percent of 1850 is: 1850(0.25) = 463 calories
- 463 of my total daily calories would come from fat
- There are 9 calories per 1 gram of fat, so 463 fat calories = 51 grams of fat

Taking my fat and protein, this is where I am at:

- Total daily caloric intake = 1850
- Total daily caloric intake from protein = 800 calories
- Total daily caloric intake from fat = 463 calories

Healthy fats include things like avocados, extra virgin olive oil, nuts, seeds, nut butters, and dark chocolate.

Carbohydrates

The remaining calories would come from carbohydrates.

- 800 protein calories + 463 fat calories = 1263 total calories
- 1850 BMR calories – 1263 protein and fat calories = 587 carbohydrate calories
- There are four calories per gram of carbohydrate, so 587 carb calories = 147 grams of carbohydrates

Healthy carbohydrates include bananas, sweet potatoes, root vegetables, berries, whole grains and oats, quinoa and of course pasta and bread.

Overall Breakdown

- Total daily caloric intake = 1850 calories
- Total daily protein intake = 1 gram per pound of body weight, which = 800 calories (200 grams of protein)
- Total daily fat intake = 25 percent of total caloric intake, which equals 463 calories (51 grams of fat)
- Total daily carbohydrate intake = remainder of calories after fat and protein is calculated, which = 587 carb calories (147 grams of carbohydrates)

Broken down by percentages:

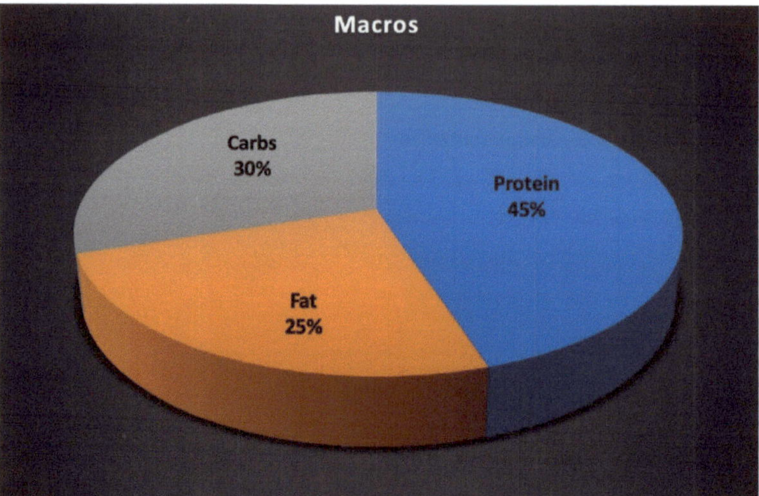

My macro breakdown

From here, you can finetune it further if you desire. Some gym rats may decide to go 45% protein, 20% fat, and 35% carbs. It's just a matter of personal preference. Once you start losing weight, you will need to re-run this calculation and update the percentages based on your new bodyweight just as a mechanism to keep it finetuned to your needs.

Intermittent Fasting

Now, if you are like me when I started, I was freaking out. I weighed 230 pounds, so I clearly enjoyed my large meals. I saw that 1,800 calories was essentially a little more than one of my everyday meals. So the next challenge I had was figuring out a way to eat only 1,850 calories per day without losing my mind. My solution to this problem was intermittent fasting.

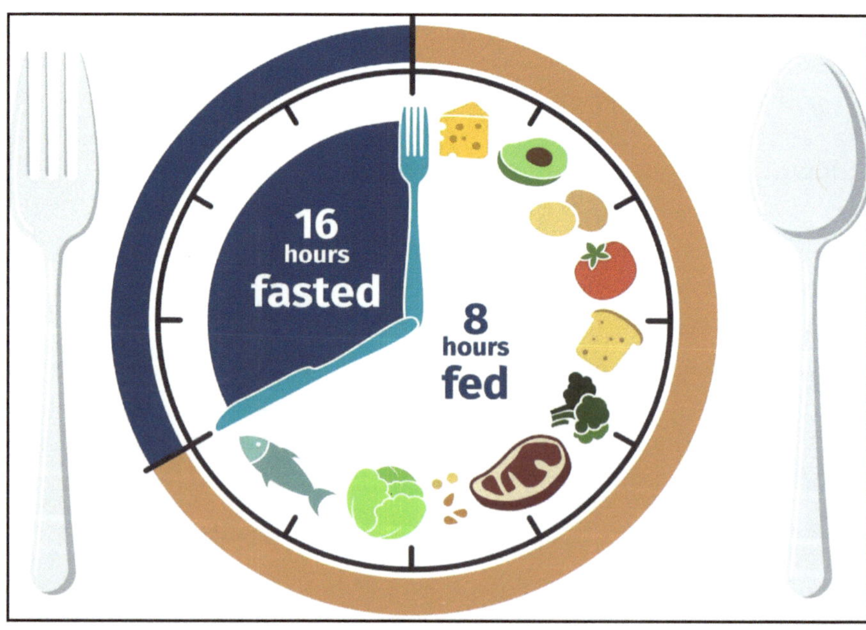

Intermittent fasting has been popular for a few years now and is a useful tool to add to your toolbox. In its simplest form, intermittent fasting is an eating pattern where you cycle between periods of eating and fasting. It does not say anything about which foods you eat, but rather when you can eat them. We already fast every day when we go to sleep at night, so intermittent fasting is a mechanism that allows us to extend the fast before we eat our breakfast meal. You can set the allowable window for eating to accommodate whatever works best for you, so I set mine at eight hours and set my times for eating from 11 am to 7 pm. My rationale was that by eating only within this eight-hour window, I could consume two 700 calorie meals, one at 11 am, and the other at 7 pm, and still have a 400 calorie snack in the afternoon.

It took me a few weeks to get used to it, but I found it much easier to maintain my diet once I did. I also added the majority of my carbs at the end of the day because that was when I was craving simple sugars, and the carbs in my diet met that need sufficiently for me to resist the urge to eat everything in sight. I also used my NLP techniques to talk myself off the ledge a few times. On the nights I did fail, I just made it a point to get back on the wagon the next day.

Set Point Theory

If you ever feel like your body hovers around a certain number on the scale, no matter how much you clean up your diet or ramp up your workouts, it's not all in your head. It is a real thing! Chances are you may be able to lose five or ten pounds only to see it creep back up within a few months of reaching your goal. Why? This is what is referred to as "set point theory." Set Point Theory stipulates that there is a biological control method in humans that actively regulates weight towards a predetermined set weight for each individual. This may occur through the regulation of energy intake or energy expenditure. This is why so many people regain weight within 3-5 years after a "successful" dieting attempt. The small minority of people that keep it off are statistical outliers. Usually, they succeed because they made such a substantial change to their life that fitness became an ingrained programmed habit.

Set Point Theory

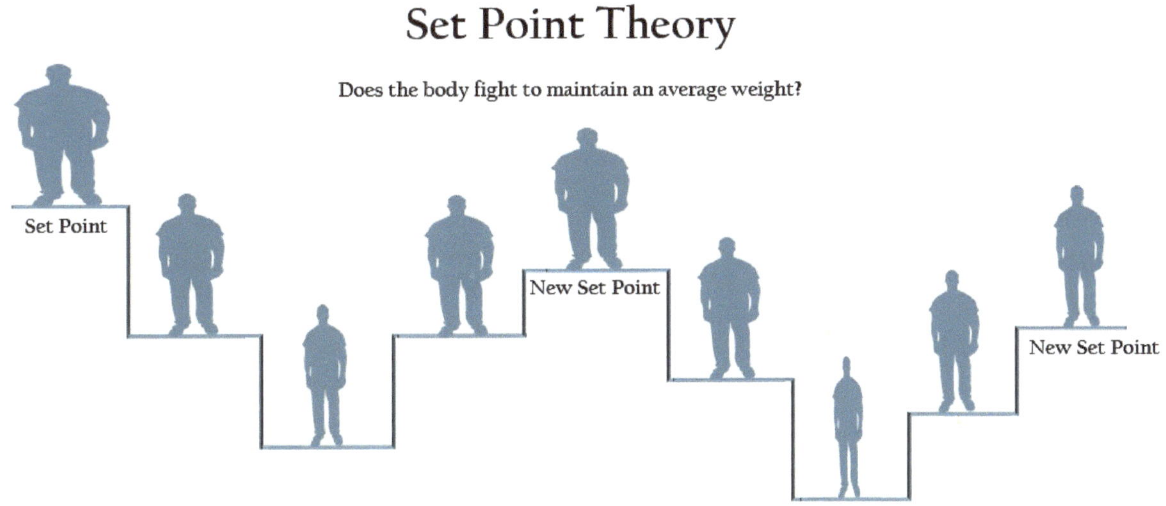

According to Set Point Theory, your body will allow you to lose or gain anywhere from five to twenty pounds, but then it will regress to your average weight over time. That is because that weight is your set point, and your body will fight to maintain it. But over time, as we age, we continue to consume the same amount of calories we did when we were younger and more active. These excess calories are stored as fat, and if we keep them on long enough, our set point moves higher, and this new weight becomes our new range from which we will hover.

This means that you will have to fight for about a year to maintain it once you reach your target weight. This is why tracking the food and macros have to become an ingrained part of your lifestyle. If you stop tracking your macros and the data, you will surely start reverting to your old miserable self. Don't! Make this a permanent lifestyle change!

Resumption of Normal Caloric Intake

Once you reach your body fat percentage goals, you will want to resume regular caloric intake. However, the time you spent in a caloric reduction mode has slowed your metabolism. So to keep in fine-tune with your body, you will want to increase your caloric intake gradually. I recommend recalculating all your metrics: BMR, TTDE, Body Fat, etc., and re-baselining your daily caloric consumption goals for maintaining your current weight. Then take your current caloric consumption and add in 50-100 calories per week. Do this over a series of weeks until you return to regular maintenance consumption goals, but keep an eye on the data to see what occurs with your weight.

Vacations & Time Off

If you go on vacation or need to take a much-needed break to unwind with family and friends, enjoy life. It is ok to eat like everyone else for a week or two. The worst damage you could do would be to gain 5-10 pounds. The key here is to get back on your program as soon as you return, and maybe dieting for a week or two to get back to your new normal state.

Key Takeaways

This chapter is about dialing your diet into a set of numbers, also referred to as macros. Success will continue as long as you are committed to the process and a large part of that success will revolve around your willingness to capture and track the data accurately. As I said at the beginning, it doesn't matter what you choose to eat, so long as you do so within the confines of your allotted macros. To do this, you must:

- Calculate your Basic Metabolic Rate (BMR) with the Harris-Benedict Equation
- Baseline your Total Daily Energy Expenditure (TDEE)
- Reduce your TDEE by 250-500 calories per day to lose fat
- Set your macros by calculating your protein needs first at 1 gram per pound of body weight, fats second at 20-25%, and filling in the remaining calories with carbohydrates

This chapter also discussed how intermittent fasting could reduce the number of meals by reducing the time frame allowed for eating to 6-8 hours. Doing so will let you eat larger meals, which is one of the main factors I contributed to my overall success and has allowed me to remain on the long haul program.

We also covered Set Point Theory, which explains why your body hovers around a set range of weight, and why it gravitates back towards that weight after successful dieting attempts. This reset makes you feel like a failure and contributes to a sense of low self-esteem. This is not a bad thing but does explain why you have to make this change a permanent part of your programming if you want to lose weight and keep it off. NLP is a useful tool that can aid you in this endeavor.

In the last part, we discussed the resumption of regular caloric intake upon reaching your goals. I recommend increasing your daily caloric intake by only 100 calories per day for a few weeks at a time, tracking the data to see how it impacts your weight. I also recommended taking some time off while on vacation to enjoy family and friends, but ensuring you have a plan in place before you go to resume your program immediately upon returning.

The next chapter covers how my process unfolded. It was a bumpy ride for me because I was developing this process through trial and error, and then dialing it in. You have the benefit of a refined process that should only need minimal tweaking for your personal preferences and lifestyle. The last chapter walks you through setting up your program.

CHAPTER FIVE: MY JOURNEY

Becoming a champion is not an easy process. It is done by focusing on what it takes to get there and not on getting there. — Nick Saban

I wanted to share my experience with this process as it unfolded. Doing data science for a large law enforcement organization has taught me a lot about data and the scientific method. Some people may argue that I am just following a comprehensive set of tried and true methods, and others may say that what I am doing has nothing to do with data science or even analysis. Data science is related to data mining, machine learning, and big data. So in the strictest sense of the term, it may be more in line with data analysis, but my point is this: It is all about the data. My experience has demonstrated to me time-after-time that success would hinge on the quality of the data that I had to analyze and drive my decisions. I placed a heavy emphasis on that and committed to following best practices, standardization, and ensuring the integrity of the data over this process. It may not always be pretty or make you proud, but it is honest and will help you along your way. Data tracking is now a part of my life process that I follow religiously to know why I look the way I look and know exactly what I need to do if I want to change it.

For your process to be successful, you need a greater understanding and awareness of how your body interacts with the food you eat. The only way to do that is through analysis of correlated data points that you track religiously. In this chapter, I will show you how I refined my process over time and the focus I placed on the data. The data I used to make changes to my process, consistently tracked my caloric intake and macros. I used a handful of measures to gauge progress: current weight, the amount gained/lost for two reporting periods (upon waking up Saturday and Tuesday mornings), body fat percentage, the circumference of my gut at its broadest point, the percent reduction in the stomach, muscle mass percentages, and body mass index. If my metrics and measures were not trending in the direction I desired, I would adjust the caloric intake and macros to get it moving in the right direction again.

I did not use any fancy tools for tracking these measures. I used a tape measure for the circumference measurement, a digital scale with an app I purchased for around $30, and an Excel spreadsheet. I understand that these scales are not as accurate as many desire, but they do give you a good baseline to begin from, and they are consistent. So while the body fat percentage may not be scientifically accurate, it is consistent, and you will see changes in it over time as you progress. Once dialed-in, you can use the mirror as your compass.

January-March

My journey began on New Year's Eve 2019. I had hit a low and decided I needed a change. The year prior, I had tried low carb dieting. Still, I didn't want to be bothered with tracking my calories, so after listening to several Audible authors say that with a low carb diet, you can consume as much as you need to feel satisfied, I did so and the results were disappointing. I was not gaining any more weight, but I wasn't losing it either. I also incorporated a journal and started writing down everything I ate and listening to the Tony Robbins program on weight loss. Tony suggested the journal for awareness, and it was useful, but while I tried the NLP concepts described in the program, they alone were not enough. This went on for the first three months of the year, and I was miserable, and it showed in all aspects of my professional and personal life. Then on March 25th, I went to a medical clinic for a severe sinus infection. While there, the nurse asked me to step up on the scale.

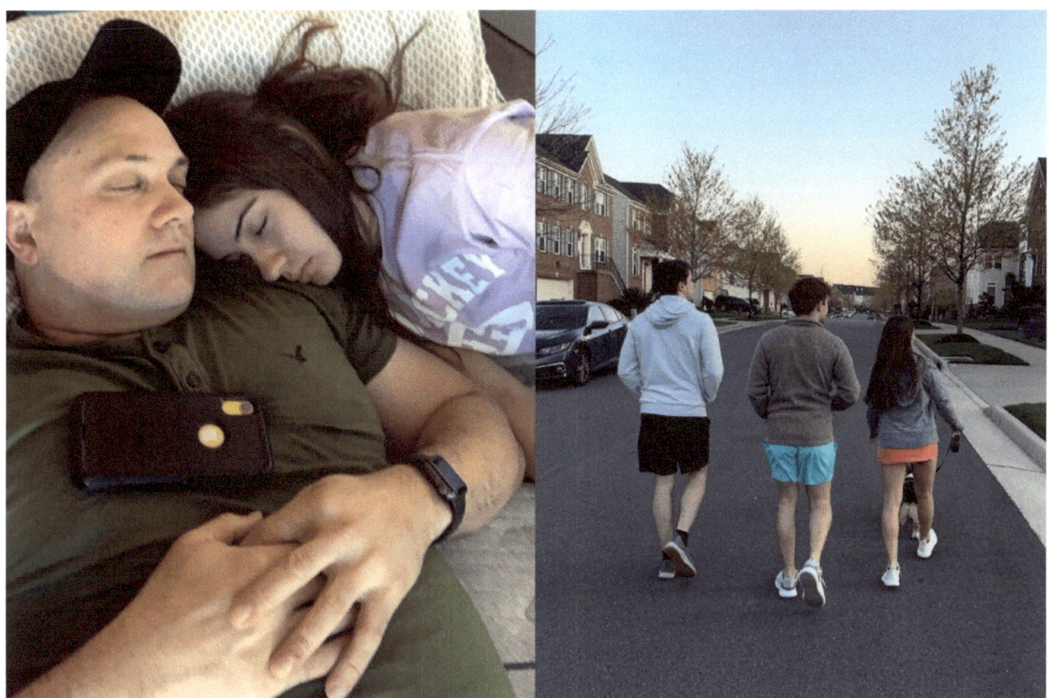

First three months of process at 225 pounds, napping and getting steps with my kids.

I didn't own a scale at the time because I had bought into the mantra that weight doesn't matter and that I should focus on what I see in the mirror. So in my mind, when I saw myself in the mirror, I thought I was a little heavy, but still in the 210-215 pounds area. So hopefully, you can imagine the shock and pain I felt when I stepped on the scale and it registered 230 pounds. I was devastated. The denial I had been in was swept away by reality. I went home and took off my shirt, but I still didn't look that bad in the mirror. So I took my phone out and snapped a few pictures, and then reality set in….I looked disgusting. It was clear that I needed to change my approach. For the first three months of the year, I logged my foods in a diary and used NLP. This was only good for five pounds. My weight went from 230 pounds to 225 pounds. This wasn't very reassuring, so I started reassessing my process.

April-June

In the second quarter of the year, I was still motivated, but lacking in progress. I knew this was a critical time because if I did not see progress soon, I would become fatigued and risk giving up. I lost no weight in April, my body fat was at 35 percent, and my gut's circumference was 45 inches. While I was discouraged with the lack of progress, I wasn't ready to throw in the towel just yet. I went to my local running store and purchased a pair of running shoes. The manager there recommended a great app, Couch to 5K, to get me running again. I used it for several weeks, but then I just started using my process of running for one song and walking one. I did this for April and found it did not cause any knee pain, but I ran slowly. My daily step goal was 15,000 steps, which was achieved by taking a run or walk in the morning and another walk in the evening. I had switched from manually logging my meals to using MyFitnessPal, and I set the goal to lose one pound per week. To do so, it set my daily caloric intake, based on my sex, height, weight, and activity levels, at 2,200 calories per day.

May was a little better than April as I saw my weight drop from 225 to 221. I was pleased to have reached my one pound a week goal, but I did not feel confident in my gains or my ability to hold on to them. However, some critical refinements made in May would go a long way towards my overall success.

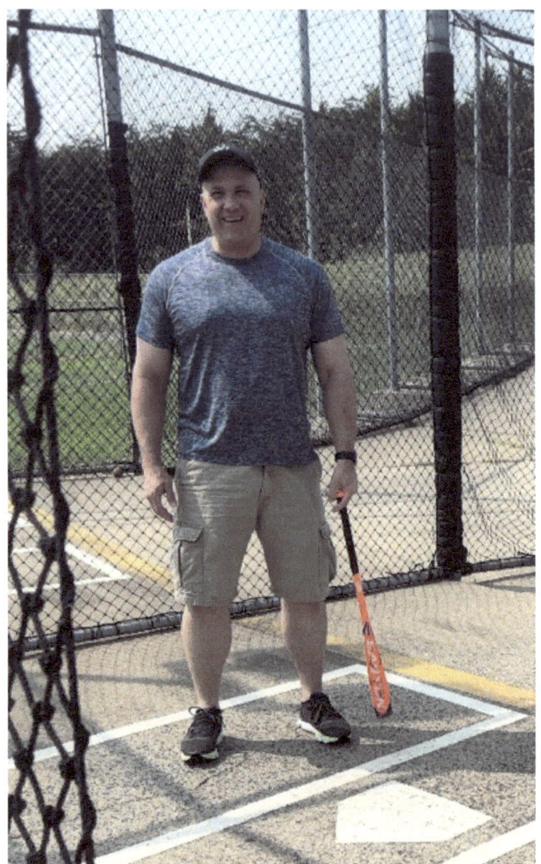 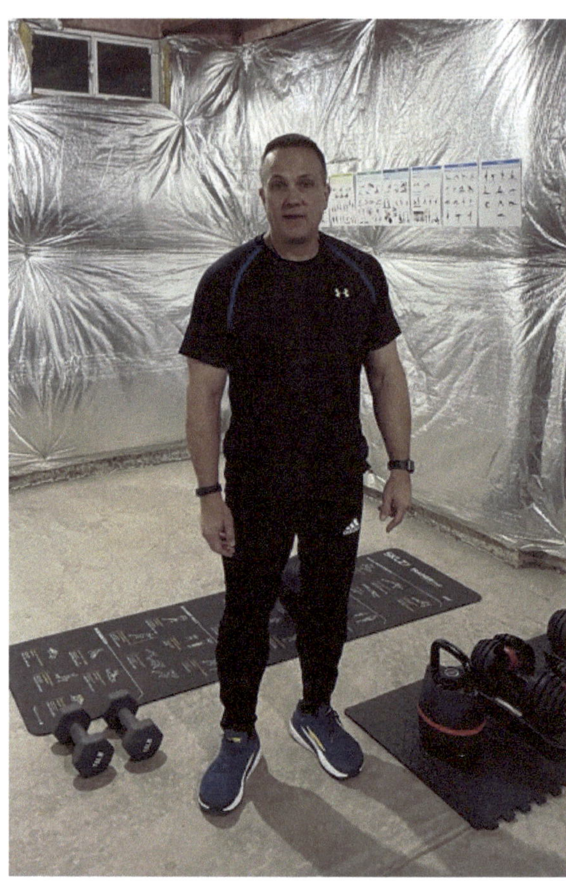

Before and after photos: 230 pounds in Summer 2019 versus 190 pounds in December 2020

The first refinement I did was dropping my caloric intake down to 1,800 calories per day. The second refinement was turning off the mechanism that compensates for exercise calories burned. There were two dynamics at play here. Initially I dropped my calories down 1,800 calories per day, but the MyFitnessPal app compensated for exercise. So if I walked 15,000 steps, it would take the 1,800 calories I burned just by breathing, add on my TDEE calories, which put me at about 2,200 calories per day. Then it would add on the calories I burned walking so that I could eat 2,500 calories and theoretically still be in a calorie deficit. However, I was not losing weight. So I researched the issue and found this addition of calories to your total is a common problem that prevents fat loss. So by setting my calories at 1,800 and turning the compensation off for exercise, I ensured that my body was operating on only my BMR calories. If you haven't turned this feature off yet, trust me, and do it right now! It will make a huge difference in the results.

I found only consuming 1,800 calories a bit challenging, but my son solved this issue by recommending I do intermittent fasting from 11 am to 7 pm. This took a few days to get used to, but it works like a charm. I consume 700 calories at 11 am, have another 400 in the afternoon, and a 700 calorie meal right at 7 pm. Initially, I woke up hungry a few times, but played around with it and found that consuming the bulk of my carbs at night allows me to sleep soundly. If the thought of intermittent fasting scares you, don't let it. I don't see it as skipping breakfast. I see it as extending my overnight fast by three additional hours before breaking it at 11. All that talk about breakfast being the most important meal is hogwash.

With the reduction in calories, I had to start planning my meals; otherwise, I would get some intense carb cravings in the evening. I've said it before, and I will repeat it; the mind is a mighty force that is not looking out for your best interest. It seeks pleasure and it isn't considering how that short-term pleasure is causing you longer-term pain. NLP helps, but the best defense is to have a planned meal ready to go. I also bought no calorie, no sugar salad dressing, and would make myself a large salad with nothing but greens, bell peppers, onions, spices, and a few nuts. The greens have few calories, and I would pack my gut with them to keep me feeling full and satiated. It works!

Then I upgrade my subscription to MyFitnessPal from free to premium. This gave me access to several dynamic features not available in the free version, and I was so fed up and desperate that I was willing to try anything. The premium version eliminated ads and allowed me to customize calorie goals, set fixed calorie intake by days of the week and each meal. You have access to an incredibly large database of foods for improved tracking. But the most appealing feature is the ability to export CSV files to my computer to analyze the data (I do work in data science, so hopefully you can see why this was so appealing.).

June was an okay month, but because I am in law enforcement, the riots that engulfed the nation threw everything out of whack. I was working crazy hours in the heat and sweating, and sometimes the meals were erratic, so planning and sticking to the diet was challenging. I was moving a lot, and that allowed me to keep burning calories. My weight dropped to 218.2. It was only about three pounds, but it was progress. My gut was down to 42 inches, which was a 3-inch drop since January. It wasn't a solid month, but I was happy I did not lose ground.

July – September: The Process Came Together

Once you see results, it becomes an addiction. – Author Unknown

I had been at this since January, and to be honest, I did not feel I had a lot to show for it. I had a determination to figure this out, and thanks to the grace of God, I never gave up. I attribute my greatest breakthrough to my good friend, Albert Herrera. Call it fate, luck, destiny.....or whatever you want, but on July 5th, Albert walked in and with a few off-handed comments, completed the process equation for me. Without even realizing it, his off-handed suggestions would make the process kick into overdrive when combined with everything else I was doing, forever changing my physical and mental outlook on life.

We discussed my weight loss journey and explained that I had made good progress, but that I felt the process was missing something. I told him that I thought I was doing everything right and focused on burning more than I consumed. I began questioning him about his diet, and the way he ate. Since Albert is always in top shape, I listened closely. Albert discussed portion control, but then he off-handedly mentioned how he tracks his macros. I stopped him and asked him to explain that part, and he discussed tracking his macro-nutrients and asked if I had been doing that. At first, I wanted to say that I had, but as I reflected on it, I had not. I had only been tracking it in terms of fat or carb with a focus on eating fewer carbs and more fat. Albert disagreed with these notions and told me I needed to focus heavier on my macros AND he said that I needed to eat MORE carbohydrates, not less. I countered with all the low carb diets floating around, and he pointed out that carbs have four calories per gram, where fats have nine. From a pure grams perspective, you could eat twice the carbs and get the same result. Albert was the lean one in the conversation, so I told him I would research the issue.

That afternoon I went to a few of the sites Albert said he frequented and read up on some of the research discussing how tracking your macros is a useful tool for monitoring your weight. It is undeniable that tracking your macros is the prominent focus bodybuilders use when trying to get lean while maintaining muscle mass. Preparing for a bodybuilding contest means they have to dial in the macros to the gram. When I read this, it hit me as entirely logical and incredibly intuitive. I was perplexed how I had missed that, but it got lost in all of the dieting fads marketing, and I overlooked it and had discounted its importance. At this point, I figured I had nothing to lose but fat, so I would try it. After tinkering around with it, I incorporated the strategy outlined in this book.

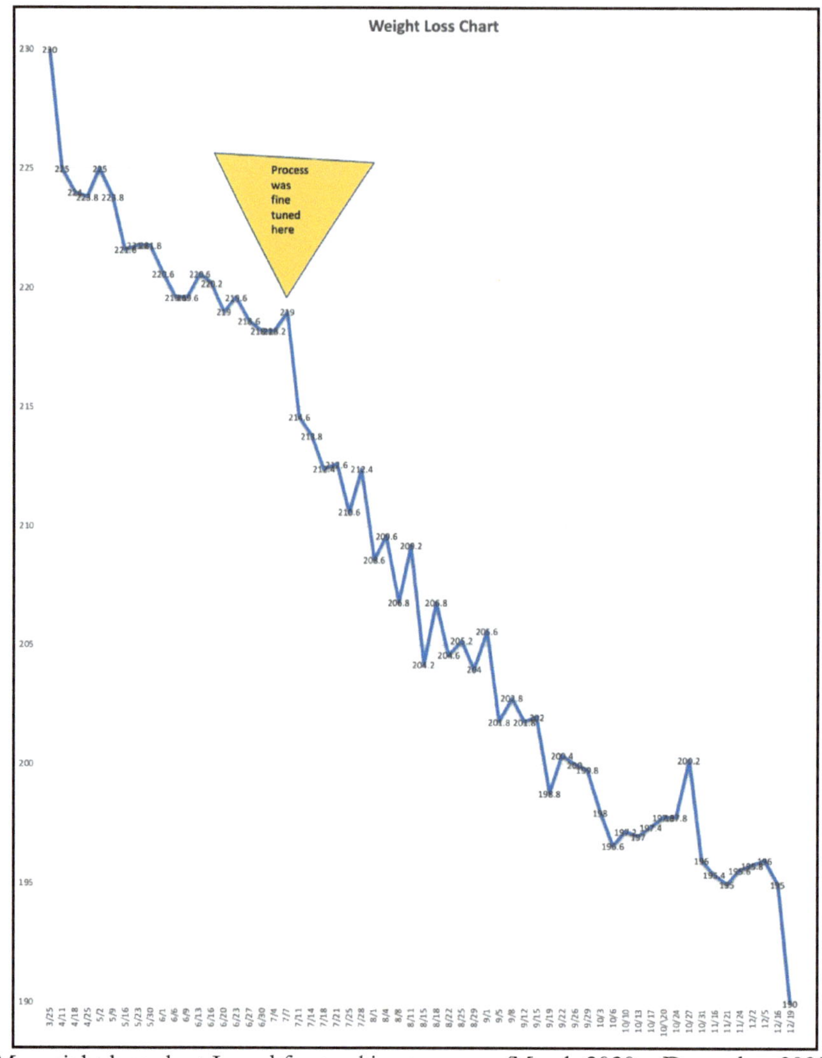

My weight loss chart I used for tracking progress (March 2020 – December 2020)

I incorporated macros on a Tuesday. To assist with this adjustment to my process, I upgraded my measuring cups and incorporated a food digital food scale to ensure I was eating proper portions. When I weighed in that Tuesday morning my weight had spiked back up to 220. I was devastated. I had been at this for almost seven months and had been doing everything I thought was right short of just outright starving myself. It was incredulous to me that a person's only option for losing weight was starving or surgery, but that was how I felt.

With my new macro strategy in hand, I started tracking my macros over the next five days. I found out quickly that this made following my diet even more crucial because my allocation of fats and carbs could be rapidly expended. I also found I had to consume large amounts of lean fish and chicken to reach my protein goals. I was so focused on this aspect that I didn't see a change. When I woke up Saturday morning, I laid in bed with a sense of anxiety for the weight in. I visualized myself getting on the weight scale and reading 220 pounds, or worse, 222! I played the week back over in my head and verified that I had done everything as outlines, so I got out of bed and approached the scale. I stepped on it and waited for the blow. The scale came back with a mind-boggling 212.4 pound reading! I almost passed out!

In the five days since I had begun tracking macros, the fat immediately started melting away! I struggled to lose ten pounds over the previous seven months and in five days, dropped seven and a half pounds. My gut circumference was at 40.5! I was running through the house screaming and yelling, "I did it! I did it! I figured it out!" My kids thought I was bonkers, but expressed disbelief at the amount of fat I lost that week. I was re-energized and ready to attack the next week with a vengeance!

The following weeks did not register as much fat loss as the first, but the results we astonishing. By the end of August, my running was improving as I got lighter, and I dropped another eight pounds. I was down to 204! My gut had crossed the threshold of 40 inches, and my body fat was now down to 18.1% (it was almost 35% eight months prior).

September showed continued progress, but I did get stuck at 204 for a few weeks. I think I was experiencing diet fatigue and was having trouble sticking to my allotted 1,800 calories. But I made a breakthrough with persistence, and I ended the month at 198 pounds, and my gut was now at 37 inches.

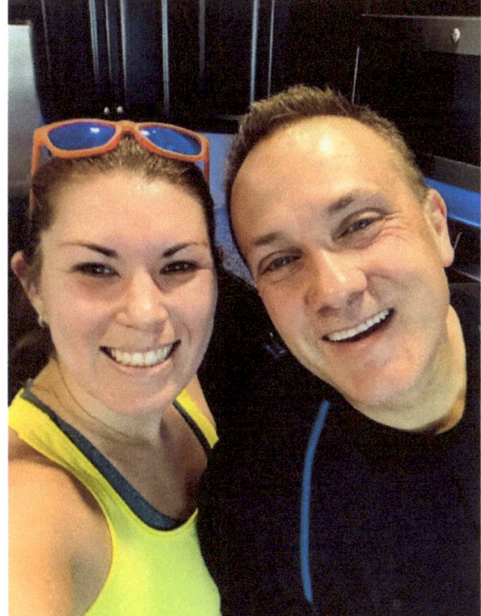

Ashley and I running to Duck Donuts as a reward

October – December

October saw my first fall as a runner in years, and it was absolutely amazing! I also continued making progress towards my goals. However, there is some truth to the adage that the last ten pounds are the hardest to lose. I was ten months into this and somewhat fatigued of consuming a low calories diet. It was never painful, but it was uncomfortable, and at times difficult to maintain. I consoled myself with the mantra that 'I didn't get this fat overnight', so I couldn't expect to lose the weight overnight either. Every day I said to myself 'This fat ain't gonna to lose itself' and I motivated myself to continue. With the last ten pounds towards my goal in sight I dug down deep and committed to making it by the end of October, or early November.

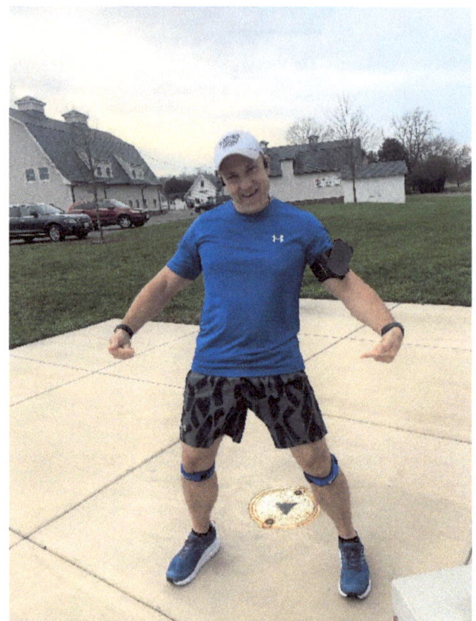

Me goofing off before a 5.5 mile run.

I moved to a new house in November and the chaos that ensued caused a setback. The good thing was that the setback did not lead to an increase in weight, but rather a pause in weight-loss. At the end of November I was at 195 pounds. I finally hit 190 in December, and based on the mirror, I believe that I am now closer to at my ideal weight for my current muscle mass. Although my journey is only beginning, I feel great!

Key Takeaways

My only goal in this chapter was to give the reader some perspective of the challenges I faced in figuring everything out. Developing this process has been rewarding, but it was incredibly frustrating, and at times I did feel hopeless. You will experience these emotions. However, you do not have to repeat the mistakes I made and get after some solid results reasonably quickly. I failed to make any progress in the first three months. I did utilize NLP techniques and did change my eating habits; however, at the time, I was not accurately tracking the data. Accurately tracking the data is critical to your success! The awareness was good, but I was fooling myself on how many calories I was eating with what I thought were proper portion sizes. From March through June, I did a better job tracking my calories, but I was still not making progress. I was moving 15,000 steps per day, yet progress was slow. When I started weighing and measuring my portion sizes and dialed in the macros, I saw the success I was seeking. Then the weight started coming off quickly. I am not going to say it was easy, because it was challenging to maintain the diet, and I did fail now and then, but I stayed on course for a majority of the time, and that carried me through. I now feel confident that I know my metabolism and can enjoy life and all it has to offer, to include food, while successfully maintaining my weight by simply turning the dials on my diet.

CHAPTER SIX: DEVELOPING YOUR PROCESS

In this chapter we are going to develop your own personal "process" for weight loss. This development will entail framing the problem, setting goals, and then objectives that support these goals. It is the basic planning process that will be tailored to fit into your daily life and programmed through repetition to become an ingrained lifelong habit. Once we are done, you will have a detailed, actionable plan that you can implement immediately. The only part I don't get into detail on is NLP and your exercise programs. Why? Mainly because NLP is a personal decision, you have to make to pursue, and only if you feel you need it. I needed it! But not everyone needs it. Some people have an incredible amount of willpower and don't struggle with a lack of discipline regarding diet. And your exercise program is based on what you like to do. As long as you are setting a move goal, whether it be a calorie burned or step goal, you set and ensure you meet your requirements. There is no one size fits all weight program, so I feel you should do one you enjoy. The only requirement is that you maintain a progressive increase in intensity constantly increasing weights and repetitions.

Step 1: Frame the Problem

Framing is a way of structuring or presenting the problem or issue. Framing involves explaining and describing the context of the problem to gain the most understanding and self-awareness. The way you frame the problem should reflect your attitude and beliefs. I also believe you should see it as it is, but not worse than it is. When framing the problem, you should be specific about:

What is the issue? For me, it was an inability to maintain a disciplined diet.

What are your issues?

What contributes to the problem? For me, it was a lack of planning, lack of a clear understanding of how my body's metabolism functions, and how I lose weight.

What contributes to your problem?

What contributes to the solution? For me, it was a clearly defined process that had specific, actionable steps that were outlined for when and how I would take them, and data-supported decisions.

What would contribute to your solution?

Once you have framed the problem by identifying the issues, what contributes to these issues, and what would contribute towards a solution, you will set your goals. Your goal is the end state metrics and measures you aim to achieve at the end of the journey. Reaching these goals is critical to being a success.

Step 2: Develop a Vision

While framing the problem I asked you to see it as it is, but not worse than it is. Now I want you to see it how you want it to be, or in other words, your vision.

What is your vision for your physical self? Here is the one I developed for myself:

> *I will be and look physically fit. I will be confident and self-assured of my appearance, and a role model for others to emulate. Monitoring my weight and adjusting my lifestyle weekly will be a habit that I desire to do.*

What is your vision?

Step 3: Set Your Goals

In setting your goals, they must be S.M.A.R.T. Goals, which means they will be:

- Specific
- Measurable
- Attainable
- Relevant
- Time-Bound

This process has a heavy focus on empirical data, which should be relatively easy to do. Here is my goal for losing weight when I began this journey:

I want to lose 40 pounds of fat while maintaining my muscle mass. I will lose at a minimum one pound of fat per week, and I want to achieve this weight within twelve months from my start date.

Once achieved, I will maintain my new weight for twelve months, making it my new set points.

Write your goals here:

Step 4: Supporting Objectives

Your objectives are those specific, actionable things you must achieve in support of reaching your goals. These will entail action steps, which is essential because action leads to motivation!

Ensure you have the tools that will support success

Having the right tools in the tool box will go a long ways towards success. Here are some recommended tools (check off once verified):

_______ Walking/running shoes
_______ Measuring cups
_______ Food scale (for weighing portion sizes)
_______ Blender, knives, cutting boards
_______ Tape measure
_______ Weight scale that tracks weight, BMI, body fat percentage (at a minimum)

Recommended (check off once verified):

______ Walking or running tools to support your move goals (Apple Watch / Fit Bit)
______ Fitness tracking apps (Strava)
______ Food log that tracks diet and macros (like MyFitnessPal)
______ Habit tracker (I purchased "Productive Habit Tracker" from the Apple App Store)
______ Music app to play tunes while exercising

Baseline Start Date

This is the official kickoff to your journey! Check off when each as they are captured.

______ Take a picture with data and time stamp and repeat every two weeks on Saturday
______ Weigh yourself and record every Saturday and Tuesday upon wakening
______ Capture the measurements you want to track and record each Saturday immediately upon awakening. For me, this was my gut. I followed my gut because it was what disgusted me the most

Exercise Regiment

<u>Move Program</u>

Your move program could be walking, running, or a combination of both. Many people also enjoy biking, hiking, and rowing but since those require additional investment or travel, I stuck to what would be easiest to incorporate into my daily life. I recommend setting either a daily target step goal or a move calorie goal. Most apps will allow you to do either. Also, I don't give specific recommendations because this journey is about finding out what works for you. I can say that I started with an initial step goal of 15,000 steps per day, and then eventually converted over to a 1,000 move calories per day. Both encompassed my walking, running, and normal daily activities. If I was not at or near my goal in the evening, I would walk after dinner to catch up.

Daily step/calorie goal: _________________

This has to be done every day. There are no days off from this. None! Not until you complete the journey.

<u>Weight Lifting Program</u>

A weight lifting program is not required but highly recommended. It will make you feel better, and muscle burns more calories. Muscle tissue is more metabolically active than fat tissue, thus building muscle just adds to the goal of weight loss. I listed my weight program in Chapter 3, and as you can see, it is a straightforward and basic program. Yet, I was able to increase my strength substantially while losing fat. I also believe the appearance of muscle covered by fat is motivating, which will drive you harder. There are a number of weight programs you can find just searching the internet, find the one that works best for you. Ashley prefers the runners strength training program that builds muscle for her to run faster and longer, everyone's program will be different. The best advice I can give is to find a program you enjoy doing and whether you go all out or just do a few sets, do something because it will contribute to your journey. Feeling strong becomes something that makes you physically and mentally more driven.

Weekly weight workout goal:____

You need to depict how many workouts you will do and estimate the time it will take. For instance, my workout takes approximately 30 minutes, and I do each body part twice a week. I combine my exercises by one half of my body during the first workout and the other half during the second. I do each of these twice a week for a total of four. I record each set, weight, and reps, and progressively work to increase with the weight or reps with each workout on at least one set for each exercise.

Calculating Macros

Remember, while it is true that losing weight is as simple as burning more calories than you consume, it is much more challenging than it sounds. If you disagree, go to any store or supermarket and look around, and you will see what I mean. Mathematically, to lose one pound of fat per week, you must burn 3,500 more calories than you consume. This equates to 500 calories per day. If you shoot for half a pound per week, it is 250 calories per day. If you go with 250 calories, you need to make sure you accurately calculate the number of calories you are consuming. Step 5 quantifies your macros.

Calculate Basic Metabolic Rate (BMR)

Your BMR is the number of calories required to keep your body functioning while at rest. It is the foundational calculation we will use to determine your daily calorie requirements. We will use the Harris-Benedict Equation formula for calculating yours. This calculation is in the Excel sheet that can be found on my webpage: www.rodneywashburn.com.

| Women | BMR = 655 + (4.35 x weight in pounds) + (4.7 x height in inches) - (4.7 x age in years) |
| Men | BMR = 66 + (6.23 x weight in pounds) + (12.7 x height in inches) - (6.8 x age in years) |

Your BMR = ____

Calculate Total Daily Energy Expenditure (TDEE)

TDEE is calculated by taking your BMR and multiplying it by the appropriate activity factor based on your lifestyle:

Sedentary (little or no exercise)	Calorie Calculation = BMR x 1.2
Lightly active (light exercise/sports 1-3 days/week)	Calorie Calculation = BMR x 1.375
Moderately active (moderate exercise/sports 3-5 days/week)	Calorie Calculation = BMR x 1.55
Very active (hard exercise/sports 6-7 days a week)	Calorie Calculation = BMR x 1.725
Extra active (very hard exercise/sports & physical job or 2x training)	Calorie Calculation = BMR x 1.9

Calculate your TDEE:

TDEE = BMR x Activity Level (either 1.2, 1.375, 1.55, 1.725, or 1.9)

TDEE = ______________________

This is what your daily calorie level where you maintain your current weight.

Daily Calorie Target for Fat Loss

With your TDEE calculated, now all we have to do is shave off either 250 calories per day or 500 calories per day. It all depends on how fast you want to lose fat. Both are doable, but 500 calories per day are more demanding than 250. Both will work so long as you are accurately capturing your caloric consumption, and remember that 250 calories do not give you a lot of room for error.

Daily calorie target: TDEE – 500 (or 250) = You daily calorie consumption

Calculate you daily calorie target: ____________

Step 5: Setting Your Macros

Macros are the secret sauce of the process. Calories track quantities, but macros highlight the quality of the foods you eat. Research shows that you are forced to make healthier food choices by monitoring macros, which will accelerate the weight loss process. We can accelerate your fat loss by properly configuring your macros. You will need to re-calculate the total calorie amount each week as you lose weight, and while the total amount of each macro will change during the process, the percentages will not.

Protein

To maintain muscle mass while losing fat, you want to consume, at a minimum, 1 gram of protein per pound of body weight. You will need to re-calculate this amount each week as you lose weight.

- Example body weight = 200 pounds
- 200 pounds x 1 gram of protein = 200 grams of protein
- Each gram of protein has 4 calories
- 200 grams of protein x 4 calories = 800 calories

Calculate your grams of protein you will consume daily:

Pounds of body weight x 1 gram of protein:

________________x_1_=____________

# of grams of protein x 4 calories = total calories from protein:

________________x_4_=____________

Fats

I recommend having fat make up 20-25% of your daily calories. I determined the grams of fat I needed daily by using the following equation:

Fat = 25 percent of daily caloric intake:

Daily caloric intake = __________

Multiply your daily calories by either 0.20 or 0.25 = total fat calories per day:

__________x_0.25_=____________

There are 9 calories per 1 gram of fat, so divide your fat calories by 9 = total grams of fat:

__________/ 9 = __________

Carbohydrates

Taking your fat and protein, this is where you are at:

Total daily caloric intake = __________

Total daily caloric intake from protein = _________

Total daily caloric intake from fat = _________

The remaining calories would come from carbohydrates.

_______ Protein calories + ________ fat calories = _________ total protein and fat calories

_______ Total daily calorie intake - ________ total protein and fat calories = ________ total carbohydrate calories

There are 4 calories per gram of carbohydrate, so _______ carb calories x 4 = _______ grams of carbohydrates

Overall Breakdown

Total daily caloric intake = _________ calories

Total daily protein intake = 1 gram per pound of body weight, which = _______ calories (_______ grams of protein)

Total daily fat intake = 25 percent of total caloric intake, which equals _______ calories (_______ grams of fat)

Total daily carbohydrate intake = remainder of calories after fat and protein is calculated, which = ______ carb calories (______ grams of carbohydrates)

Broken down by percentages:

Protein = ____%
Fat = ____%
Carbohydrates = _____%

Over the next few weeks you can fine tune your macros based on the amount of weight loss.

Step 6: Intermittent Fast & Meal Planning

Intermittent fasting can be tailored to what works for you. I found success by fasting from 7 pm each night until 11 am the next day. I never deviated from this.

Sub-Objective 1: Establish Fasting Hours

I will fast from ________ until ________ each day.

Every Sunday is meal prep day. This is critical to your success. Don't wing it. Make a methodical well thought out plan.

Key Takeaways

This chapter is arguably the most crucial of the entire book. These baselines are not exact but serve as excellent starting points. Once you calculate your baselines and set your goals, you can begin capturing and tracking the data to see how your body responds. Your success hinges on your willingness to properly capture all of the foods you consume and then make adjustments to your overall caloric intake based on the results. Committing to this will get you in sync with your metabolism to add of drop weight as desired. The control this gives you over your weight and life is liberating and gives you a sense of self-confidence to accomplish anything you pursue.

CONCLUSION

I wrote this book because of my frustrations with weight-loss. In my research, I found a lot of either ambiguity about weight loss or a drastic oversimplification of the issue. The ambiguity is by design because the weight-loss industry is a billion-dollar business. It allows the industry to push a constant stream of books and products that supposedly support weight-loss, but never provide a clear and concise process that individuals can permanently incorporate into their daily lives. The oversimplification of the matter comes from those who say that it's a basic math equation that says that you must burn more than you eat if you want to lose weight. While this is factually correct, it is much more difficult to action than stated.

My analysis of success repeatedly found that there is usually a well-defined process at the heart of the problem, and all of its operations revolve around it. This focus on process is found in organizations like Amazon, the University of Alabama's football program, Wal-Mart, Google, and the Home Depot, to name a few. Sustained success comes from focusing on these processes and continuously making improvements to them. It is for that reason that I felt weight-loss should be approached in the same manner. Then the challenge was finding the right information that would get directly to the heart of the matter. It took me some time and effort, but I feel you now have that process that you can action to make the changes you want to your weight.

If you have tried losing weight before and failed, it isn't because of a lack of willpower. It is how you communicate with your brain in this area of your life. This failure to properly communicate is why two people can come from the same backgrounds, have the same opportunities, and yet one will achieve much greater success than the other. If several people can be programmed to do something well, then the program can be replicated in someone else. This replication is what neuro-linguistic programming (NLP) is all about. To develop a sound process, you need to find several people who excel at what you want to model. The commonalities in their methods can be replicated and reprogrammed into your strategy for success.

You also need to ensure you have the supporting tools that support the process. These supportive tools include measuring cups, tape measures, weight scales, and apps for your data collection and metrics. These support tools are vital to your success. Without them, you will not be able to ensure that you are eating the appropriate portions or accurately capturing your data. None of these supporting tools are expensive, and all are worth the investment. Supportive tools also include exercise gear like running or walking shoes or any other equipment to make attacking your move goals a more enjoyable experience.

Your exercise routine is a personal matter, but I believe that it should entail both resistance training and movement goals. The transition from a sedentary lifestyle to an active one can induce anxiety, but over time will become the most enjoyable part of your day. You will need to set a minimum move goal requirement in either steps or calories burned. How you achieve them through running, walking, or hiking is totally up to you.

The book's diet section will allow you to dial your diet down to the empirical numbers of calories and the percentages of those calories that are to be carbohydrates, fats, and proteins. The proper combination of these macronutrients is a powerful fat loss accelerator. Once dialed in, it will sometimes feel like the fat is melting away in front of your eyes from week-to-week. The baseline calculations will not be exact but will be close. Starting from these baselines will allow you to dial the calories up or down as needed to achieve your stated goals. Accurately capturing and tracking the data will get you in near-perfect sync with your metabolism. This understanding alone is life-changing if applied in a meaningful way! I also shared my journey in sufficient detail so that you could fully understand how I came to this process. The process development provided will allow you to set your own SMART goals for your roadmap to success.

Lastly, I wanted to say a sincere thank you for reading my book. It truly means a lot, and I hope you find the information useful and applicable to your own life and goals. I set up www.rodneywashburn.com to gather feedback so that I can improve the process as we advance. I also ask that you leave a book review on Amazon.com. Thank you! Good luck! Don't give up! Stay committed! You have everything you need here to achieve the results you desire. All you need to do now is take massive action. So go forth and conquer your goals and objectives!

ACKNOWLEDGEMENTS

I want to start out by thanking Amazon Publishing for empowering the people to self-publish and sell to a global audience.

This book wouldn't have been possible without the mentorship of the analysts, data scientists, researchers, engineers, academics, co-workers, and other professionals that taught me how to develop and test insight-related ideas in my own research projects over the last twenty-plus years.

I want to give a special thanks to my co-workers that debated some of the theories and concepts I analyzed during this journey. Albert Herrera for his contributions on "macros," and Dane Hammack for his views on calculating the Basic Mass Index.

I owe an enormous debt of gratitude to those who gave me detailed and constructive comments on one or more chapters, including Dane Hammack, Kelly Washburn, Luis Tafoya, Kate Pattison, and Ashley Hoffman. They gave freely of their time to discuss nuances of the text and pushed me to clarify concepts, explore particular facets of insight work, and explain the rationales for specific recommendations.

I'm also immensely grateful to my children, Lance and Kayla, for allowing me to transform our kitchen into my own personal learning laboratory during my endless hours of meal prepping. I cannot express my gratitude enough for being able to share this transformative research experience with you. I hope you learned something about your own metabolism while enduring this process with me. If any part of this has a positive long-term impact on your health, then it was well worth the time and effort.

My mom and dad for all you have ever done for me. Without a doubt, I won the birth lottery. I know I didn't make it easy on you and my career choices always caused you concern, but rest easy now knowing that your thoughts and prayers were heard by Him, and it all turned out alright.

Finally, I want to thank my soon-to-be wife, Ashley, for being my trusted companion in running, dieting, and life. A lifelong partner makes both the journey and destination worthwhile. I appreciate your patience and I love you more than you will ever know.

ABOUT THE AUTHOR

Rodney Washburn sees the world as a set of data problems and finds fulfillment in solving them. His projects are derived from this concept. Rodney served five years in the Marines and then twenty-five years as a senior leader with a large federal law enforcement organization where he currently has oversight of all data science operations. He holds a Master's Degree from the Eisenhower School for National Security and Resourcing Strategy. Rodney is an expert in law enforcement operations, law enforcement intelligence, data analytics, gap analysis, and requirements development. He currently resides in Northern Virginia with his fiancé and children.

Rodney can be found on:

- Facebook
- Instagram
- Twitter
- Linked In
- Amazon.com
- Website: www.rodneywashburn.com

DOWNLOADS

I added an Excel book as a companion to this short book to assist you with outlining your goals and objectives, and quantifying you calories and macros. You can download this companion Excel sheet at my site: www.rodneywashburn.com.